PHARMACY TECHNICIAN

FLASH REVIEW

PHARMACY
TECHNICIAN
FLASH REVIEW

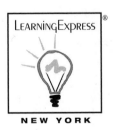

LearningExpress®

NEW YORK

Cataloging-in-Publication Data is on file with the Library of Congress.

Printed in the United States of America

9 8 7 6 5 4 3 2 1

First Edition

ISBN 978-1-57685-960-5

For information on LearningExpress, other LearningExpress products, or bulk sales,
please write to us at:
    80 Broad Street
    4th Floor
    New York, NY 10004

Or visit us at:
    www.learningexpressllc.com

CONTENTS

INTRODUCTION

Pharmacy technicians are vital components of the healthcare team. They can work in a variety of settings, including hospitals, retail pharmacies, long-term care facilities, home healthcare and infusion pharmacies, and even nuclear and compounding pharmacies. Each setting offers a chance for a pharmacy technician to demonstrate different levels of abilities and knowledge. Regardless of the location, most states require pharmacy technicians to be certified. This book can help prepare you for the Pharmacy Technician Certification Exam (PTCE).

About the Pharmacy Technician Certification Exam

The PTCE is offered by the Pharmacy Technician Certification Board (PTCB) and is a nationally accredited exam. Applicants who pass the exam are then designated as certified pharmacy technicians (CPhT). The certification must be renewed every two years, and 20 hours of continuing education is required for renewal, with at least one of those hours being in the subject of pharmacy law.

The exam is comprised of 90 multiple-choice questions, 10 of which are questions that will not be scored and are placed randomly throughout the exam. These questions will not affect your score. The time allotted to complete the exam is one hour and fifty minutes, and the test is administered on a computer.

The PTCE has recently been updated after a job analysis study, with nine new knowledge domains that are organized to better assess technician competencies. The following table lists the new knowledge domains and shows the percentage of content of the PTCE devoted to each section.

Knowledge Domain	Percent of PTCE Content
Pharmacology for Technicians	13.75
Pharmacy Law and Regulations	12.5
Sterile and Nonsterile Compounding	8.75
Medication Safety	12.5
Pharmacy Quality Assurance	7.5
Medication Order Entry and Fill Process	17.5
Pharmacy Inventory Management	8.75
Pharmacy Billing and Reimbursement	8.75
Pharmacy Information Systems Usage and Application	10

About the Exam for the Certification of Pharmacy Technicians

The ExCPT is a nationally accredited exam offered by the National Healthcareer Association. Applicants who pass the exam are designated as certified pharmacy technicians (CPhT). This certification must be renewed every two years, and during this period the CPhT must complete at least 20 hours of continuing education, including at least one hour of Pharmacy Law.

The exam is taken on a computer and contains 110 questions, 10 of which are pre-test questions that will not be scored. You will have two hours to complete the test. The questions that are scored cover three general knowledge areas:

Knowledge Area	Percent of ExCPT Content
Regulations and Technician Duties • General technician duties • Controlled substances • Laws and regulations	25%
Drugs and Drug Therapy • Drug classification • Most frequently prescribed medications	23%
The Dispensing Process • Prescription information • Preparing/dispensing prescriptions • Calculations • Sterile products, unit dose, and repackaging	52%

About the Book

This book contains more than 600 concepts, terms, math equations, and skills to help prepare you for the PTCE. It is divided into sections that follow the new layout of the PTCE for easy studying. The top 200 drugs are included in easy-to-study chart format for easy learning, and sample math problems are included for extra practice.

This book should not be memorized in one sitting! Instead, set aside time each day to review and practice terms. Quiz yourself periodically, and move forward from concepts when you have mastered them. Keep a positive attitude, and stay focused. Becoming a certified pharmacy technician is not easy, but the end result is worth the hard work.

Good luck!

PHARMACY TECHNICIAN

FLASH REVIEW

METRIC SYSTEM

. . . .

HOUSEHOLD SYSTEM

. . . .

Common metric conversions encountered for weight and volume:

Weight:
Kilogram = kg
Gram = g
Milligram = mg
Microgram = mcg

Each row represents an equivalent weight (e.g., 1 kg = 1,000 g)

1 kg	1,000 g	1,000,000 mg	1,000,000,000 mcg
	1 g	1,000 mg	1,000,000 mcg
		1 mg	1,000 mcg

Volume:
Liter = L
Milliliter = mL

Each row represents an equivalent volume (e.g., 1 L = 1,000 mL)

1 L	1,000 mL

· ·

Common household conversions encountered for volume and weight:

Volume:
Tablespoon = T
Teaspoon = tsp

Each row represents an equivalent volume (e.g., 1 gallon = 128 fl oz)

1 gallon	4 quarts	8 pints	16 cups	128 fl oz	256 T	768 tsp
	1 quart	2 pints	4 cups	32 fl oz	64 T	192 tsp
		1 pint	2 cups	16 fl oz	32 T	96 tsp
			1 cup	8 fl oz	16 T	48 tsp
				1 fl oz	2 T	6 tsp
					1 T	3 tsp

Each row represents an equivalent weight

1 pound	16 ounces

· ·

APOTHECARY SYSTEM

. . . .

CONVERSIONS BETWEEN AND WITHIN MEASUREMENT SYSTEMS

. . . .

The apothecary system is an older, less frequently used, system of measurement. The most common units in this system are:

1 grain	65 mg
1 dram	5 mL

. . . .

Household Measurement	Metric Measurement
1 oz	30 g
1 lb	454 g
2.2 lb	1 kg
1 tsp	5 mL
1 T	15 mL
1 fl oz	30 mL
1 cup (8 fl oz)	240 mL
1 pint (16 fl oz)	480 mL
1 quart (32 fl oz)	960 mL

When converting between metric units align your units from biggest to smallest.

kg	g	mg	mcg

When you move from a unit that is bigger (kg) to smaller (g), you will always move the decimal point to the right. When you move from a unit that is smaller (g) to bigger (kg), you will move the decimal point to the left. In the chart above, each unit is separated by three decimal places. To convert from kg to g, move the decimal point to the right three places. To convert from mcg to g, move the decimal point to the left six places.

Example: Convert 5 kg into mg: Look at the chart—mg is 2 blocks to the right of kg, which means we will move our decimal point 6 places to the right: 5 kg = 5,000,000 mg.

. . . .

ROMAN NUMERALS

. . . .

MILITARY TIME

. . . .

MATH PRACTICE

Roman Numeral	Value	Roman Numeral	Value	Roman Numeral	Value
I	1	VI	6	XX	20
II	2	VII	7	L	50
III	3	VIII	8	C	100
IV	4	IX	9	D	500
V	5	X	10	M	1,000

Three main rules for Roman numerals:

1. A letter repeated once or twice is added that many times, but never more than 3 (XXX = 30, MM = 2,000).

2. When a letter placed after another letter is smaller than the previous letter, the two are added together (VII = 7, XI = 11, LV = 55).

3. When a letter placed before another letter is smaller than the following letter, the value of the first letter is subtracted from the value of the second letter (IV = 4, IX = 9, XL = 40).

· ·

Military time is used frequently in the hospital system for calculation of administration times.

Standard Time	Military Time	Standard Time	Military Time	Standard Time	Military Time
1:00 A.M.	0100 hours	9:00 A.M.	0900 hours	5:00 P.M.	1700 hours
2:00 A.M.	0200 hours	10:00 A.M.	1000 hours	6:00 P.M.	1800 hours
3:00 A.M.	0300 hours	11:00 A.M.	1100 hours	7:00 P.M.	1900 hours
4:00 A.M.	0400 hours	12:00 P.M.	1200 hours	8:00 P.M.	2000 hours
5:00 A.M.	0500 hours	1:00 P.M.	1300 hours	9:00 P.M.	2100 hours
6:00 A.M.	0600 hours	2:00 P.M.	1400 hours	10:00 P.M.	2200 hours
7:00 A.M.	0700 hours	3:00 P.M.	1500 hours	11:00 P.M.	2300 hours
8:00 A.M.	0800 hours	4:00 P.M.	1600 hours	12:00 A.M.	0000 hours

· ·

PHARMACY TECHNICIAN FLASH REVIEW

DOSAGE CALCULATION EXAMPLE

. . . .

DAY SUPPLY

. . . .

One way to solve dosage calculations is to use the **ratio-proportion** method to calculate the amount of medication to give. This method requires two ratios that are set to an equal proportion.

- Example: A patient needs to take a 250 mg dose of a medication, and the pharmacy stocks 125 mg/5 mL. How much volume should be dispensed?

Start with what you are looking for and make this your x. We are looking for volume, which in this case equals mL. Now put this unknown over your dose—we are trying to find the volume that goes with the dose that was ordered.

$$\frac{x\,mL}{250\,mg}$$

We now have our first ratio, and we can set it equal to our second ratio, which is the stock concentration of the drug, 125 mg/5 mL. It is important that the same units are in the numerator (top of the ratio) and in the denominator (bottom of the ratio).

$$\frac{x\,mL}{250\,mg} = \frac{5\,mL}{125\,mg}$$

To solve, we simply cross-multiply and divide. To do this, multiply the two diagonal values from the x (250 and 5) and then divide by the last value (125):

$$(250) \times (5) \div (125) = 10\ mL\ or\ 2\ teaspoons\ dose$$

. . . .

The number of days a medication should last when used correctly is important to determine for insurance purposes and refill restrictions.

Steps to solve:

1. First, determine how much will be taken in one day.
   a. Calculate this step by multiplying the dose by the frequency of administration.
2. Next, divide the total quantity being dispensed by the amount taken in one day.

Example: Take 1 tab PO TID dispense #30

Step 1. Determine how much in one day: 1 tab × 3 = 3 tabs

Step 2. Divide the quantity dispensed by the amount taken in one day: 30 ÷ 3 = 10

This prescription is a 10-day supply.

. . . .

PERCENT ERROR

. . . .

UNITS

. . . .

Used in compounding to determine the amount of error when a substance may have been weighed or measured inaccurately.

Calculated as follows:

Step 1. Calculate the amount of error by subtracting the two values (ignore if a negative number results).

Step 2. Divide this amount by the exact value, or the value expected to be obtained.

Step 3. Convert this to a percentage by multiplying this decimal by 100 or moving the decimal place two places to the right.

Example: You are to dispense 500 mg of a powder. The first measurement taken is 500 mg, but when a more accurate balance is used, you determine the measurement to be 505 mg. What is the percentage of error?

Step 1. Find the amount of error = 505 − 500 = 5

Step 2. Divide this by the exact value (500) = 5 ÷ 500 = 0.01

Step 3. Convert to percent by multiplying by 100 = 0.01 × 100 = 1% error

. . . .

Examples of medications measured in units:

- insulin
- heparin
- penicillin

Insulin is always 100 units in 1 mL and generally comes in a 10 mL vial.

Calculations are completed in the same manner.

Example: If a patient requires 35 units of insulin, how many mL will be injected?

Set up the ratio. We are looking for mL, so that is our x.

$$\frac{x \text{ mL}}{35 \text{ units}} = \frac{1 \text{ mL}}{100 \text{ units}}$$

Cross-multiply and divide: (35)(1) ÷ 100 = 0.35 mL to be injected

. . . .

PHARMACY TECHNICIAN FLASH REVIEW

MILLIEQUIVALENTS (mEq)

. . . .

CONCENTRATIONS AND DILUTIONS

. . . .

Units used to measure electrolytes—the strength of an ion in a medication

Examples of medications measured in milliequivalents:

- potassium chloride
- sodium
- phosphate

Calculations are completed in the same manner.

Example: If a patient is to get 25 mEq of potassium, and the pharmacy stocks a 40 mEq/mL vial, how much should be injected into the patient?

$$\frac{x\ mL}{25\ mEq} = \frac{1\ mL}{40\ mEq}$$

Cross-multiply and divide: (25)(1) ÷ 40 = 0.625 mL to be injected

· ·

A concentrate is a drug that must be diluted prior to administration. A diluent is an inactive substance added to the concentrate to lower the concentration of the final solution.

To calculate, use a simple formula: $C_1V_1 = C_2V_2$

C_1 = the concentration of the stock

V_1 = the volume of the stock used

C_2 = the concentration of the final product

V_2 = the volume of the final product

Example: You are making 1 L of a 0.7% solution. You have a stock of 15% solution to use. How much stock will you need to make this product?

C_1 = the concentration of the stock = 15%

V_1 = the volume of the stock used = x

C_2 = the concentration of the final product = 0.7%

V_2 = the volume of the final product = 1,000 mL

Multiply the two known values and divide by the remaining value to solve for the unknown.

(0.7)(1,000) ÷ 15 = 46.7 mL of stock

To determine the amount of diluent you will need, simply subtract this value from the final volume:

1,000 mL – 46.7 mL = 953.3 mL of diluent

· ·

TEMPERATURE CONVERSIONS

. . . .

PERCENT STRENGTH

. . . .

When converting from Celsius temperature to Fahrenheit, use the following formula:

$$°F = (1.8 × °C) + 32$$

When converting from Fahrenheit temperature to Celsius, use the following formula:

$$°C = \frac{°F - 32}{1.8}$$

• •

The concentration of a drug or active ingredient (**solute**) dissolved in a vehicle (solvent) expressed as a fraction, ratio, or percentage.

Example: A 5% solution can be written as 5/100, 5:100 or 0.05.

• •

ALLIGATIONS

Alligations are used when a prescriber orders a medication in a strength that the pharmacy does not have, and the pharmacy must compound the order from two stocks—one of higher strength and one of lower strength than the desired concentration.

Example: Make 200 mL of a 5% solution using 2.5% and 10% stock solutions. How much of each will you need?

Start with a tic-tac-toe.

10		
	5	
2.5		

Place the highest concentration (10) in the upper left square, the desired concentration (5) in the middle square, and the lowest concentration (2.5) in the lower left square, keeping the values in their percentage form.

10		2.5
	5	
2.5		5

Next, subtract the center number from the upper left value (10 – 5) and place this value in the lower right square. Than subtract the lower left square from the center (5 – 2.5), and place this value in the upper right square.

2.5		2.5
	5	
2.5		5

Next, add the upper and lower right (2.5 + 5) corners to determine total parts.

2.5 + 5 = 7.5 total parts

To determine how much of each strength, read across from the percentage:

For the 10%: read across to 2.5, so there are 2.5 parts out of 7.5 total. To determine what quantity of the total volume this is, set up a ratio-proportion:

$$\frac{x \text{ mL}}{200 \text{ mL}} = \frac{2.5}{7.5} = 66.7 \text{ mL}$$

Do the same process for the 2.5% stock solution. Read across to the 5 = 5 parts out of 7.5 total. To determine what quantity of the total volume this is, set up a ratio-proportion:

$$\frac{x \text{ mL}}{200 \text{ mL}} = \frac{5}{7.5} = 133.3 \text{ mL}$$

WEIGHT/WEIGHT (W/W)

....

WEIGHT/VOLUME (W/V)

....

VOLUME/VOLUME (V/V)

The number of grams of a drug in 100 g of final product.

Example: A 2.5% cream has 2.5 g of drug in 100 g of product.

We can use this ratio to determine how much active ingredient would be in a given quantity.

Example: How much active ingredient is in a 45 g tube of 2.5% cream?

Remember: 2.5% w/w = 2.5 g/100 g

$$\frac{x\,g}{45\,g} = \frac{2.5\,g}{100\,g}$$

Cross-multiply and divide: $(45)(2.5) \div 100 = 1.125$ g of drug in a 45 g tube of 2.5% w/w cream

· ·

The number of grams of a drug in 100 mL of final product.

Example: A 2.5% solution has 2.5 g of drug in 100 mL of product.

We can use this ratio to determine how much active ingredient would be in a given quantity.

Example: How many grams of active ingredient are in 500 mL of a 23% solution?

Remember: 23% w/v = 23 g/100 mL

$$\frac{x\,g}{500\,g} = \frac{23\,g}{100\,mL}$$

Cross-multiply and divide: $(500)(23) \div 100 = 115$ g of drug in 500 mL of 23% w/v solution

· ·

The number of milliliters of a drug in 100 mL of final product.

Example: A 2.5% solution has 2.5 mL of drug in 100 mL of solution.

We can use this ratio to determine how much active ingredient would be in a given quantity.

Example: How many milliliters of IPA are in 250 mL of a 70% solution?

Remember: 70% v/v = 70 mL/100 mL

$$\frac{x\,mL}{250\,g} = \frac{70\,mL}{100\,mL}$$

Cross-multiply and divide: $(250)(70) \div 100 = 175$ mL of IPA in 250 mL of 70% v/v solution

IV FLOW RATES

. . . .

IV DRIP RATES

. . . .

IV flow rates are based on a measured amount given per unit of time. To calculate, the volume of the infusion and the amount of time of the infusion must be known. Simply divide the volume by the infusion time to determine the rate:

$$\frac{\text{Volume of infusion}}{\text{Infusion time}} = \text{infusion rate}$$

Example: If a 1,500 mL IV is infused over 5 hours, what is the infusion rate?

$$\frac{1,500 \text{ mL}}{5 \text{ hours}} = 300 \text{ mL/hr}$$

To calculate the time of infusion when the rate and volume are known, simply take the volume of the infusion and divide it by the rate:

$$\frac{\text{Volume of infusion}}{\text{Infusion rate}} = \text{infusion time}$$

Example: If a 1,500 mL IV is infused at a rate of 300 mL/hr, what is the time of infusion?

$$\frac{1,500 \text{ mL}}{300 \text{ mL/hr}} = 5 \text{ hours}$$

· ·

Drip rates are calculated in drops per minute. There are different **drop factors** that each IV set will be labeled with. Some examples are 15 gtt/mL or 20 gtt/mL, and a microdrip comes as 60 gtt/mL.

To calculate gtt/min:

$$\frac{(\text{Total volume}) \times (\text{drop factor})}{\text{Total minutes}}$$

Example: If a patient has a 500 mL order for 4 hours and a drop factor of 20 gtt/mL, what is the drip rate?

First, convert hours to minutes: 4 hours × 60 minutes = 240 minutes.

$$(500)(20) \div 240 \text{ min} = 4 \text{ gtt/min}$$

· ·

BUSINESS MATH

. . . .

Discount: a reduced price

To calculate: purchase price × discount rate (percent as a decimal) = discount

Purchase price – discount = new discounted price

Example: Discount = 25%, purchase price = $100, $100 × 0.25 = $25

$100 – $25 = $75 = **new discounted price**

Markup: the difference between the selling price and the purchase price

To calculate: Find difference between selling price and purchase price.

To calculate the markup rate, divide the markup by the purchase price (cost) and multiply by 100 to get a percent.

Example: Purchase price = $10, selling price = $22, difference = 22 – 10 = **$12 = markup**

Markup rate = 12 ÷ 10 × 100 = **120% markup rate**

Overhead: the sum of all expenses of running a pharmacy, including utilities, drugs, salaries, and so on.

. . . .

MEDICATION ORDER

. . . .

ADMISSION ORDER

. . . .

STAT ORDER

An order written by a prescriber for a patient in a hospital or other inpatient setting.

. . . .

A type of medication order written by a physician if a patient should be admitted into the hospital; this order is sometimes written when a patient has visited the emergency room and, after a physician's assessment, it is decided he or she should be admitted into the facility.

Will contain:

- drugs the patient is currently taking

- drugs the patient should continue taking

- new medications the physician has ordered for the patient

- lab tests ordered, and any results obtained while in the ER

- suspected diagnosis

- any allergies

- weight and height of patient (for dosing)

- medical record number

- room number

. . . .

A type of medication order sent to the pharmacy that must be filled immediately.

DISCHARGE ORDER

. . . .

PRN ORDER

. . . .

UNIT DOSE

A medication order that gives instructions for a patient who is being discharged from the hospital; it should include all at-home information and prescription instructions for the patient until follow-up with a primary care physician can occur.

· ·

A medication order given on an "as needed" basis for specific signs and symptoms exhibited by a patient; some examples of symptoms requiring a PRN medication could be:

- fever

- pain

- anxiety or restlessness

- itching

- coughing

- sneezing

· ·

A drug used in a hospital or other inpatient setting that is prepackaged from bulk for a single administration for one patient.

Benefits of unit dose are:

- easy for nurse dispensing to patients

- cuts down on medication errors (each unit dose may be bar-coded)

- less waste of medication

UNIT DOSE LABELS

. . . .

FLOOR STOCK

. . . .

AUTOMATED DISPENSING CABINETS

To be repackaged from bulk, the labeling of unit doses must contain specific information:

- drug name (generic or brand)

- strength of medication

- name of original manufacturer

- original lot number and expiration date of manufacturer (for tracking in the event of a recall)

- bar code

- facility expiration date—cannot exceed date given by manufacturer

. . . .

Drugs that are stored on each unit of the hospital that are frequently prescribed for that unit; most floor stocks are stored in automated dispensing cabinets.

. . . .

A secure storage device that contains medications used by specific patient care units; access is limited to authorized individuals who have patient orders that need to be filled.

Examples of ADCs:

- Pyxis® (Cardinal Health)

- AcuDose-Rx® (McKesson)

- Omnicell®

- Rx-Station® (Cerner)

- Med Select® (Amerisource Bergen)

PRESCRIPTION

. . . .

INSCRIPTION

. . . .

SIGNA

An order written for a patient by a licensed practitioner to be filled by a pharmacist.

Parts of the prescription:

- inscription

- signa

- subscription

- superscription

· ·

Part of the prescription that includes the name and strength of the medication prescribed and the amount to be dispensed.

Example: Lipitor (atorvastatin) 10 mg #30

· ·

Also known as the sig; directions to the patient.

Example: Take 1 tablet by mouth daily

PHARMACY TECHNICIAN FLASH REVIEW

SUBSCRIPTION

. . . .

SUPERSCRIPTION

. . . .

DISPENSE AS WRITTEN (DAW)

PHARMACY TECHNICIAN FLASH REVIEW

Part of the prescription that includes directions to the pharmacist for dispensing the medication.

Example: Number of refills permitted

· ·

Part of the prescription that includes the information at the top: the patient's name and address, date of birth, date the prescription was written, and Rx symbol.

· ·

A part of a prescription that when checked indicates that the generic of a drug must *not* be dispensed; brand name is required.

DAW CODES

· ·

PATIENT PROFILE

· ·

Submitted to the insurance company to determine if the proper brand name or generic medication is being dispensed.

DAW Code	Meaning
DAW 0	Default used when dispensing a generic drug or when dispensing a brand name product that does not have a generic available
DAW 1	*Prescriber* indicates dispense as written
DAW 2	*Patient* requests brand name product
DAW 3	*Pharmacist* requests brand name product be dispensed
DAW 4	Generic is not in stock, so the brand name product must be dispensed
DAW 5	Brand dispensed but priced as generic
DAW 6	Brand name is necessary: used for **prior authorization** cases
DAW 7	Substitution not allowed; brand mandated by law
DAW 8	Generic is not currently available: either not being manufactured or not being distributed
DAW 9	Other

A database of information stored in a pharmacy system for each patient; should be continually updated by the pharmacy technician.

Contains the following information:

- name
- address
- phone number
- birth date
- gender
- allergy information
- medical information (preexisting conditions or diagnoses)
- insurance information
- prescriptions filled
- preference for child-resistant containers
- may contain other preferences, such as generic substitution or large-print labels

ALLERGIES

. . . .

AUXILIARY LABEL

. . . .

PRESCRIPTION CONTAINER LABEL

Hypersensitivity of the immune system that may begin immediately after taking a medication or take weeks to show symptoms.

Examples of allergy indicators:

- rash

- watery eyes

- swelling

- itching

- wheezing

More severe allergic reactions can result in **anaphylaxis**, which leads to swelling of the airways and difficulty breathing; can lead to death if not immediately treated.

· ·

Bright, colorful label placed on a bottle label to provide information in addition to what is on the bottle label; alerts patients to specific information to which careful attention should be paid.

· ·

Label should be affixed to the medication container and match the prescription exactly. Specific information is required to be printed on the label, including:

- pharmacy name, address, and telephone number

- patient's name

- date prescription was filled

- prescriber's name

- prescription Rx number (unique to pharmacy)

- medication name and strength

- directions for use

- quantity of medication (if controlled, should be spelled out)

- expiration date

- refills allowed (if any)

- initials of pharmacist dispensing prescription

COUNTING TRAY

. . . .

TABLET SPLITTER

. . . .

SCORED TABLETS

A device used to count tablets, capsules, or other solid oral medications and transfer these dosage forms from the stock bottle to the patient's medication bottle.

- A spatula is used to count in quantities of **five**.

- A tray should be cleaned with 70% IPA after medications with a powdery residue to prevent cross-contamination of medications.

- Pharmacies may have separate trays for counting penicillin derivatives and chemotherapy agents.

· ·

A device used to split tablets in half.

· ·

Tablets that have a line or crevice to make splitting easier.

FILL PROCESS

. . . .

Process of filling prescriptions for patients in an outpatient setting:

1. Obtain prescription from the patient.

   a. if new patient, add her or him into the system

   b. if current patient, update profile with current information

2. Enter prescription information into the computer.

3. Obtain a prescription label and compare it to the original prescription to check accuracy.

4. Pull the appropriate medication from the shelf using the NDC number to confirm the correct medication was selected.

5. If medication is capsules or tablets, a counting tray will be used, and then they will be poured into an amber vial.

6. If medication is a liquid, an appropriately sized bottle should be used to pour the liquid to the proper level.

7. After proper filling, the prescription label is then affixed to the medication container.

8. The prescription must then be checked by a pharmacist for **final verification** or the **final check** before being dispensed to the patient

9. If the patient is coming back to pick up the prescription later, the medication will be filed alphabetically in a specific area of the pharmacy.

10. If the patient is waiting, the pharmacy technician can ask the patient whether he or she has any questions for the pharmacist and whether counseling is required.

Remember: A pharmacy technician must never counsel patients.

PHARMACY TECHNICIAN FLASH REVIEW

REFILLS

. . . .

UNIT-OF-USE

. . . .

EXPIRATION DATE

Refills can be easily handled by a technician when a patient calls in and refills remain on the patient profile for that medication.

Some situations require more attention:

- Early refill
    - Dosage may have changed or patient may be requiring a vacation fill—insurance company may need to be contacted

- No refills
    - A patient may be out of refills and the physician must be called for a refill authorization request
    - The prescription may be older than 12 months

- Controlled substance
    - C-II cannot be refilled
    - C-III and C-IV can only be refilled five times within a 6-month period

. . . .

Packaging provided by the manufacturer in the most commonly-dispensed unit.

Examples:

- a package of 30 tablets of a medication taken every day

- a monthly pack of birth control

- a four-pack of a medication taken once a week for one month

Pharmacy technicians can place the label directly on these packages and help minimize the case of medication errors and counting mistakes.

. . . .

The date at which a drug is no longer effective or safe to use.

PHARMACY TECHNICIAN FLASH REVIEW

PATIENT PACKAGE INSERT

. . . .

MEDICATION GUIDE

. . . .

INSTITUTE FOR SAFE MEDICATION PRACTICES (ISMP)

Required by the FDA for all medications dispensed; provides information about the drug for the patient, including:

- how the drug works
- what to do if a dose is missed
- contraindications
- warnings
- side effects
- overdose information
- dosages and packing information
- indications and use

· ·

Supplemental information required by the FDA to be included in addition to the patient package insert for specific drugs.

Examples of some medications requiring a **MedGuide** are:

- Accutane
- antidepressants
- birth control
- NSAIDs
- medications for ADD including Adderall®, Concerta®, Ritalin®, and Strattera®

· ·

An organization whose mission is to investigate medication errors and help provide error-reduction strategies to the medical community.

Has created:

- Medication Errors Reporting Program (MERP)—a voluntary reporting program
- list of unsafe abbreviations
- list of look-alike/sound-alike drugs to be dispensed carefully

LOOK-ALIKE/SOUND-ALIKE (LASA)

. . . .

TALL MAN LETTERING

. . . .

HIGH-ALERT MEDICATIONS

A list of medications developed by the ISMP that have the potential to be confused with other drugs.

An example of some are in the table that follows, the rest can be found at http://www.ismp.org/tools/confuseddrugnames.pdf.

Drug Name	Confused Drug Name
Celexa®	Celebrex®
Lamisil®	Lamictal®
Novolog®	Humalog®
Paxil®	Plavix®
Prednisone	Prednisolone
Tramadol®	Trazodone®
Viagra®	Allegra®
Xanax®	Zantac®

• •

Lettering used to help distinguish drug names that may otherwise be confused.

Example: **SERO**quel® and **SINE**quan®

For a complete list, visit http://www.ismp.org/tools/confuseddrugnames .pdf.

• •

Medications that if used in error carry a greater risk of causing patient harm.

The ISMP created a list of medications considered high risk. This can be found at http://www.ismp.org/tools/highalertmedications.pdf.

ERROR-PRONE ABBREVIATIONS

. . . .

LEADING ZERO

. . . .

TRAILING ZERO

The ISMP has created a list of abbreviations that are frequently misinterpreted. The use of these abbreviations should be limited, and if a technician encounters one in practice, he or she should always verify the correct meaning.

Abbreviation	Meaning	Mistaken for
QOD	Every other day	QD (once daily), QID (four times daily)
AD, AS, AU	Right ear, left ear, each ear	OD, OS, OU (right eye, left eye, each eye)
U or u	Unit	The number 0 or 4
$MgSO_4$	Magnesium sulfate	MSO_4 (morphine sulfate)
BT	Bedtime	BID (twice daily)

For a complete list, visit http://www.ismp.org/tools/errorprone abbreviations.pdf.

. . . .

The zero placed before the decimal point: **0**.7

A leading zero is required and should always be included in dosing.

. . . .

The zero placed after or to the right of the decimal point: 7.**0**

A trailing zero is unnecessary and, if misinterpreted, could cause a tenfold increase in a medication to be incorrectly dispensed.

PATIENT IDENTIFIER

. . . .

MEDICATION ERROR

. . . .

PHARMACIST INTERVENTION

PHARMACY TECHNICIAN FLASH REVIEW

Anything that can identify the patient when administering his or her medication.

Examples include:

- name
- identification number
- telephone number
- date of birth
- social security number
- address

• •

Any preventable event that may cause or lead to inappropriate medication use or patient harm.

Can be broken down into different types of errors:

- **Omissions Error**—a prescribed dose is due to be given but not administered
- **Wrong Time Error**—a prescribed dose is given out of the designated range of the hospital time guidelines
- **Wrong Dose Error**—a dose is given above or below the prescribed dose

• •

Some issues require the decision making and clinical knowledge of a pharmacist. The following should be done by a pharmacist and never a technician:

- counseling a patient
- OTC product recommendation
- therapeutic substitution
- discussing with patients what to do in the event of a missed dose or misuse of the medication
- final verification of medications

SYSTEMIC EFFECT

. . . .

LOCALIZED EFFECT

. . . .

ROUTE OF ADMINISTRATION

An effect of a drug that involves the entire body; for example, a blood pressure lowering agent.

· ·

An effect of a drug that involves a specific part of the body only; for example, using a numbing agent on an injured area.

· ·

The way by which a drug enters into the body; selected based on several factors, including:

• speed of onset required

• patient status (for example, ability to swallow a tablet)

• drug's absorption characteristics

ORAL (PO)

. . . .

TABLET

. . . .

CAPLET

Most common route of administration—giving a medication by mouth.

- least expensive and most convenient route

- not the quickest method because medication must be absorbed into the bloodstream from the GI tract

- achieves best rates of patient's compliance to drug therapy

. . . .

A solid dosage form made by compression.

. . . .

A solid tablet dosage form shaped like a capsule; can assist in easier swallowing of large tablets.

CHEWABLE TABLET

. . . .

DELAYED RELEASE (DR)

. . . .

ENTERIC COATED (EC)

A tablet that is to be chewed and swallowed, not swallowed whole; ideal for children and patients who have difficulty swallowing tablets; has a faster onset of action than regular tablets.

· ·

Tablets that are specially coated and designed to delay absorption and dissolving until after the drug has bypassed the stomach.

· ·

A tablet that is specially coated to aid in swallowing and to bypass the stomach so that it will not dissolve until it reaches the small intestine; designed for medications that may be harsh on the stomach (aspirin).

EXTENDED RELEASE (XR, XL)

. . . .

CONTROLLED RELEASE (CR)

. . . .

SUSTAINED RELEASE (SR)

A type of medication that allows a reduced frequency in dosing.

· ·

A type of extended-release formulation that delivers the drug at a certain rate for a specific period of time.

· ·

A type of extended-release formulation that releases the medication slowly over a specific period of time.

CAPSULE

. . . .

SOLUTION

. . . .

SOLUTE

PHARMACY TECHNICIAN FLASH REVIEW

A container, usually made of gelatin, that contains a medication to be dissolved in the GI tract; easier to swallow than a tablet and generally has a slightly faster onset of action.

· ·

A liquid in which the active ingredient is completely dissolved.

· ·

The part of the solution that is dissolved in the liquid, that is, the active ingredient.

SOLVENT

....

ELIXIR

....

SYRUP

The part of the solution that is composed of the liquid portion; the liquid that does the dissolving (water when mixed with Kool-Aid).

· ·

A liquid dosage form that is sweetened and usually contains alcohol.

· ·

A thick solution made with water and a large amount of sugar.

SUSPENSION

....

EMULSION

....

LOZENGE/TROCHE

A liquid dosage form that is composed of undissolved particles of active ingredient suspended in a liquid; patients must be told to shake well when given a suspension.

. . . .

A mixture of two substances that normally would not mix together; must be shaken well prior to use.

. . . .

A solid oral dosage form that usually has localized effects; proper use is to suck or chew lozenges (for example, troches for thrush treatment, and nicotine gum).

OINTMENT

. . . .

PASTE

. . . .

CREAM

Topical dosage form that contains more oil than water and tends to have a greasy or oily feel; a water-in-oil preparation (W/O): Neosporin®.

. . . .

Topical dosage form similar to an ointment, but it creates a heavier consistency, and thus the application is thicker than an ointment or cream: sunscreen.

. . . .

Topical dosage form that contains more water than oil; an oil-in-water preparation (O/W): hydrocortisone cream for itching.

LOTION

. . . .

TRANSDERMAL PATCH

. . . .

INTRAUTERINE DEVICE (IUD)

Topical dosage form composed of an oil-in-water base and thinner in a consistency lighter than cream, which helps them to absorb faster and be lighter on the skin: OTC moisturizers.

. . . .

Topical dosage form designed to deliver a drug enclosed within a patch to the body through skin absorption: Nitroglycerin (angina) and Duragesic® (pain—C-II).

. . . .

Small device inserted into the uterus to prevent pregnancy; effective means of birth control for several years.

PHARMACY TECHNICIAN FLASH REVIEW

ANTIBIOTICS

. . . .

BROAD SPECTRUM

. . . .

PENICILLIN

Drugs used to kill or inhibit growth of certain types of bacteria.

Two types:

• bacteriostatic—an antibiotic that inhibits the growth of bacteria

• bactericidal—an antibiotic that kills bacteria

• •

Antibiotics that are effective against a wide variety of bacteria, and effectiveness is not limited to one specific type of bacteria (gram positive or gram negative).

• •

Drug Class	Penicillin
Mechanism of Action	Prevents bacteria from forming cell wall
Indication	Otitis media, strep throat, respiratory infections, gonorrhea, and syphilis
Side Effects	Diarrhea (most common), allergy in approximately 10% of the population
Examples	• penicillin • amoxicillin • ampicillin
Hint	-cillin ending for penicillins

CEPHALOSPORIN

· ·

SULFONAMIDES

· ·

TETRACYCLINES

Drug Class	Cephalosporin
Mechanism of Action	Prevents bacteria from forming cell wall (similar to penicillin)
Indication	Upper respiratory infections, sinus infections, pneumonia
Side Effects	Diarrhea, 1% chance of cross allergies if allergic to penicillin
Examples	• cephalexin (Keflex®) • cefdinir (Omnicef®)
Hint	*cef/ceph-* beginning for cephalosporins

Drug Class	Sulfonamides
Mechanism of Action	Disrupts the pathway for producing folic acid in bacteria
Indication	UTIs, otitis media
Side Effects	Rash, photosensitivity
Examples	• sulfasalazine • sulfamethoxazole with trimethoprim (Bactrim®)
Hint	*sulfa-* beginning for sulfonamides
Special Considerations	Can cause Stevens-Johnson syndrome, a potentially fatal reaction marked by large red blotches of the skin; should take with plenty of water to avoid crystallization in urine

Drug Class	Tetracyclines
Mechanism of Action	Inhibits protein synthesis in bacteria
Indication	Acne, chronic bronchitis, walking pneumonia, Lyme disease
Side Effects	Rash, photosensitivity
Examples	• doxycycline hyclate (Vibramycin®) • tetracycline (Sumycin®) • minocycline (Minocin®)
Hint	*-cycline* ending for tetracyclines
Special Considerations	Antacids interfere with absorption and will render medication ineffective when taken concurrently; should not be given to children or pregnant women; taking expired tetracycline can cause a fatal renal disease

MACROLIDES

....

FLUOROQUINOLONES

....

Drug Class	Macrolides
Mechanism of Action	Inhibits protein synthesis in bacteria
Indication	Respiratory infections, chlamydia
Side Effects	GI distress
Examples	• azithromycin (Z-Pak®) • clarithromycin (Biaxin®) • erythromycin (E-mycin®, Ery-Tab®)
Hint	*-mycin* ending for macrolides

Drug Class	Fluoroquinolones
Mechanism of Action	Inhibits bacterial DNA replication, causing bacterial cell death
Indication	UTIs, upper respiratory infections, infectious diarrhea, bone/joint infections
Side Effects	Nausea/vomiting, dizziness
Examples	• ciprofloxacin (Cipro®) • levofloxacin (Levaquin®)
Hint	*-floxacin* ending for fluoroquinolones
Special Considerations	Antacids interfere with absorption and will render medication ineffective when taken concurrently; should not be given to children or pregnant women

AMINOGLYCOSIDES

· ·

VANCOMYCIN

· ·

Drug Class	Aminoglycosides
Mechanism of Action	Inhibits bacterial protein synthesis
Indication	Life-threatening infections
Side Effects	Nephrotoxicity and ototoxicity
Examples	• gentamicin (Garamycin®) • amikacin (Amikin®)
Special Considerations	Doses are adjusted on a patient-specific basis and measured daily to ensure no toxicity is occurring

Drug Class	Vancomycin
Mechanism of Action	Inhibits cell wall synthesis
Indication	Life-threatening infections, such as MRSA, *Clostridium difficile* (*C. Diff*), or endocarditis
Side Effects	Nephrotoxicity and ototoxicity
Examples	• Vancomycin HCl
Special Considerations	Doses are adjusted on a patient-specific basis and measured daily to ensure no toxicity is occurring (trough and peak measuring); if infused too quickly, patient will flush—known as red man syndrome

METRONIDAZOLE

. . . .

ANTIFUNGAL

. . . .

ANTIVIRAL

Drug Class	Metronidazole (Flagyl®)
Indication	Bacterial infections caused by anaerobic bacteria, protozoa infections, gynecologic infections, and as part of a multidrug regimen for *H. Pylori*
Special Considerations	Patient must be counseled to **not drink alcohol** while taking this medication—if taken with alcohol, patient will develop severe nausea and vomiting

Drug Class	Antifungal
Mechanism of Action	Kill fungal cells by exploiting key differences between fungal and human cells
Indication	Infections caused by fungus including athlete's foot, ringworm, oral candidiasis (thrush), and vaginal yeast infections
Examples	• nystatin (Mycostatin®) • amphotericin B (Fungizone®) • clotrimazole (Lotrimin®)
Hint	Many antifungal agents end in *–zole*

Drug Class	Antiviral
Mechanism of Action	Inactivate enzymes needed for viral replication
Indication	Used to treat infections caused by viruses including herpes, hepatitis, and influenza
Examples	• acyclovir (Zovirax®) • valacyclovir (Valtrex®) • famciclovir (Famvir®)
Hint	Many antiviral agents end in *–vir*

PHARMACY TECHNICIAN FLASH REVIEW

ANTIRETROVIRAL

. . . .

ANTIHISTAMINES

. . . .

ANTITUSSIVES

Drug Class	Antiretroviral
Indication	Used to treat infections caused by HIV/AIDS
Classes of Antiretrovirals	• Nucleoside Reverse Transcriptase Inhibitors (NRTIs) • Nonnucleoside Reverse Transcriptase Inhibitors (NNRTIs) • Protease Inhibitors (PIs) • Fusion Inhibitors

. . . .

Drug Class	Antihistamines
Mechanism of Action	Block histamine from working on the H_1 in the respiratory system
Indication	Used to provide relief of allergy symptoms caused by the release of histamine
Examples	• diphenhydramine (Benadryl®) • fexofenadine (Allegra®) • loratadine (Claritin®)
Special Considerations	Can cause drowsiness and should not be taken by pregnant women (crosses placenta)

. . . .

Drug Class	Antitussives
Mechanism of Action	Suppression of the cough reflex in the brain or nerve receptors along the respiratory system
Indication	Used to provide relief of cough, especially dry or non-productive coughs
Examples	• codeine • dextromethorphan (Delsym®) • benzonatate (Tessalon Perles®)
Special Considerations	Codeine is a very effective antitussive agent, but is a controlled substance for its abuse potential

DECONGESTANTS

. . . .

EXPECTORANTS

. . . .

ANTIDEPRESSANTS

PHARMACY TECHNICIAN FLASH REVIEW

Drug Class	Decongestants
Mechanism of Action	Constrict the blood vessels in the nasal passages so mucous and fluid can drain and thus alleviate the feeling of stuffiness
Indication	Used to provide relief of nasal congestion from allergies, sinusitis, and the common cold
Examples	• pseudoephedrine (Sudafed®) • phenylephrine (Sudafed PE®)
Special Considerations	Can increase blood pressure and heart rate, so should be avoided in patients with hypertension; can cause CNS stimulation. Pseudoephedrine is regulated under the Combat Methamphetamine Act, and its sale is limited to a certain quantity per month.

Drug Class	Expectorants
Mechanism of Action	Decrease thickness of mucous in lungs
Indication	Used to decrease thickness and break up fluid in the lungs so that a cough will become productive and allow the patient to expel mucous
Examples	• guaifenesin (Robitussin®, Mucinex®)
Special Considerations	Drinking water helps rid the lungs of mucous naturally

Drug Class	Antidepressants
Description of Condition	Depression is characterized by feelings of intense sadness, problems eating and sleeping, lack of self-worth, and pessimistic behavior and thoughts.
Indication	Used to treat depression
Classes of Antidepressants	• Selective Serotonin Reuptake Inhibitors (SSRIs) • Serotonin and Norepinephrine Reuptake Inhibitors (SNRIs) • Monoamine Oxidase Inhibitors (MAOIs) • Tricyclic Antidepressants (TCAs)
Special Considerations	Antidepressants have a delay of onset (usually 10–21 days) as the patient's neurotransmitters are modified from the medication, so these drugs should never be taken on an "as needed" basis; a **medication guide** must always be dispensed with all antidepressants.

PHARMACY TECHNICIAN FLASH REVIEW

SELECTIVE SEROTONIN REUPTAKE INHIBITORS (SSRI)

. . . .

SEROTONIN NOREPINEPHRINE REUPTAKE INHIBITORS (SNRI)

. . . .

MONOAMINE OXIDASE INHIBITORS (MAOI)

Drug Class	Selective Serotonin Reuptake Inhibitors (SSRI)
Mechanism of Action	Block the reuptake of serotonin, which increases serotonin levels in the brain
Indication	Used to treat depression and obsessive-compulsive disorders
Examples	• citalopram (Celexa®) • escitalopram (Lexapro®) • fluoxetine (Prozac®) • paroxetine (Paxil®) • sertraline (Zoloft®)
Special Considerations	Serotonin syndrome can occur if an SSRI is taken with another drug that increases serotonin levels in the brain—rare, but can be fatal

. . . .

Drug Class	Serotonin Norepinephrine Reuptake Inhibitors (SNRI)
Mechanism of Action	Block the reuptake of both serotonin and norepinephrine, which increases levels of both neurotransmitters in the brain
Indication	Used to treat depression and pain
Examples	• duloxetine (Cymbalta®) • venlafaxine (Effexor®) • desvenlafaxine (Pristiq®)
Special Considerations	Generally used in patients when SSRIs are not effective

. . . .

Drug Class	Monoamine Oxidase Inhibitors (MAOI)
Mechanism of Action	Block the enzyme that breaks down serotonin and norepinephrine
Indication	Used to treat depression
Examples	• selegiline (Eldepryl®) • phenelzine (Nardil®)
Special Considerations	Have many drug interactions: should not take with ephedrine, amphetamine, methylphenidate, levodopa, or meperidine; patients need to avoid aged cheeses and certain meats and vegetables; patients require a 2-week washout period after discontinuing medication before a new therapy begins.

TRICYCLIC ANTIDEPRESSANT (TCA)

. . . .

ANTIANXIETY AGENTS

. . . .

BENZODIAZEPINES

Drug Class	Tricyclic Antidepressant (TCA)
Mechanism of Action	Blocks the reuptake of serotonin or norepinephrine
Indication	Used to treat depression and bedwetting in children
Examples	• amitriptyline (Elavil®) • doxepin (Sinequan®) • imipramine (Tofranil®)
Special Considerations	Has even longer delay of onset—results may not show for weeks; anticholinergic side effects = urinary retention, dry mouth, constipation; cardiotoxic in higher doses and must be monitored

Drug Class	Antianxiety Agents
Description of Condition	Anxiety is characterized by a state of uneasiness and apprehension about possible events
Indication	Used to treat anxiety resulting from either external events or internal neurological imbalance
Examples of Antianxiety Agents	• benzodiazepines • buspirone (Buspar®)
Special Considerations	Some antianxiety agents may cause dependence and are abused—many are controlled substances

Drug Class	Benzodiazepines
Mechanism of Action	Enhance the effect of the neurotransmitter gamma amino butyric acid (GABA), which results in sedation and relaxing properties
Indication	Used to treat anxiety
Examples	• alprazolam (Xanax®) • diazepam (Valium®) • lorazepam (Ativan®)
Special Considerations	Are all schedule IV controlled substances; cause drowsiness and sedation
Hint	-am ending for benzodiazepines

HYPNOTICS AND SEDATIVES

. . . .

ANTIPSYCHOTICS

. . . .

ANALGESICS

Drug Class	Hypnotics and Sedatives
Mechanism of Action	Enhance the effect of the neurotransmitter GABA, which results in sedation
Indication	Used to treat insomnia and sleep disorders
Examples	• eszopiclone (Lunesta®) • zaleplon (Sonata®) • zolpidem (Ambien®)
Special Considerations	Work the same way as the benzodiazepines, but quicker and have a shorter half-life; benzodiazepines can also be used to treat sleep disorders, especially when insomnia is driven by anxiety-related issues

Drug Class	Antipsychotics
Description of Condition	Schizophrenia is a chronic psychiatric illness that may include delusions, hallucinations, and bizarre behavior
Indication	Used to treat schizophrenia
Mechanism of Action	Block dopamine receptors in the brain, which helps control emotions
Examples of Antipyschotics	**Atypical** • aripiprazole (Abilify®) • clozapine (Cloazril®) • olanzapine (Zyprexa®) • quetiapine (Seroquel®) • risperidone (Risperdal®) • ziprasidone (Geodon®) **Typical** • prochlorperazine (Compazine®) • haloperidol (Haldol®)
Special Considerations	Antipsychotics have very undesirable side effects, including tardive dyskinesia, which involves involuntary movements of the mouth, lips, and sometimes limbs; atypical antipsychotics are newer drugs that tend to have fewer side effects than typical antipsychotics.

Drugs that relieve pain; can be non-narcotic or narcotic (derived from opioid).

NARCOTIC ANALGESIC

. . . .

NON-NARCOTIC ANALGESIC

. . . .

OPIOIDS

PHARMACY TECHNICIAN FLASH REVIEW

Drug Class	Narcotic Analgesic
Mechanism of Action	Activate opiate receptors, which helps inhibit the pain pathway
Indication	Used to treat moderate to severe pain
Examples	• fentanyl (Duragesic®) • hydromorphone (Dilaudid®) • meperidine (Demerol®) • morphine (Kadian®, Avinza®, MS Contin®, MSIR®) • oxycodone (Oxycontin®) • oxycodone with acetaminophen (Percocet®)
Special Considerations	All are controlled substances and have high abuse potential

. . . .

Drug Class	Non-Narcotic Analgesic
Indication	Used to treat mild to moderate pain
Examples	• non-steroidal anti-inflammatory drugs (NSAIDs) • cyclooxygenase-2 inhibitors (COX-2 inhibitors) • aspirin • acetaminophen (Tylenol®)

. . . .

One of the oldest natural drugs; found in the poppy plant

• Produces a feeling of euphoria and is therefore useful in treating pain

• Can also be used for cough suppression

• Common side effects are constipation and nausea/vomiting

ANTIPYRETICS

. . . .

ANTI-INFLAMMATORY

. . . .

NON-STEROIDAL ANTI-INFLAMMATORY DRUGS (NSAIDs)

Medication that lowers a fever.

· ·

Medication that decreases inflammation.

· ·

Drug Class	Non-Steroidal Anti-Inflammatory Drugs (NSAIDs)
Mechanism of Action	Inhibit prostaglandin synthesis, which helps prevent inflammation from occurring
Indication	Used to lower inflammation and fever, and for mild to moderate pain relief
Examples	• ibuprofen (Advil®, Motrin®) • naproxen (Aleve®, Naprosyn®) • diclofenac (Voltaren®) • ketorolac (Toradol®) • indomethacin (Indocin®)
Special Considerations	Can cause GI distress due to the inhibition of prostaglandin synthesis

COX-2 INHIBITORS

. . . .

ASPIRIN

. . . .

ACETAMINOPHEN (TYLENOL)

Drug Class	COX-2 Inhibitors
Mechanism of Action	Inhibit cyclooxygenase-2 (COX-2) enzymes that are produced during inflammation
Indication	Used to help treat the symptoms of rheumatoid arthritis and osteoarthritis, and other mild to moderate pain
Examples	• celecoxib (Celebrex®)
Special Considerations	All other COX-2 inhibitors have been withdrawn from the market except celecoxib.

. . . .

Drug Class	Aspirin
Mechanism of Action	Inhibit prostaglandin synthesis
Indication	Can be used for mild pain, fever reduction, and inflammation
Special Considerations	• Should not be given to children who have been exposed to the chickenpox—can cause **Reye's syndrome** • Should not be given to patients on warfarin (Coumadin®) • Should not be taken by pregnant women

. . . .

Drug Class	Acetaminophen (Tylenol)
Mechanism of Action	Elevate the pain threshold and suppress prostaglandin synthesis
Indication	Can be used for mild to moderate pain and fever reduction
Special Considerations	• **Can** be taken during pregnancy • Does not cause GI problems, but can cause liver damage if taking over 3 g (3,000 mg) per day

ACETYLCYSTEINE (MUCOMYST, ACETADOTE)

....

MUSCLE RELAXANTS

....

DISEASE-MODIFYING ANTIRHEUMATIC AGENTS (DMARDs)

Drug Class	Acetylcysteine (Mucomyst, Acetadote)
Mechanism of Action	Attach to acetaminophen and detoxifies the metabolite
Indication	Antidote for acetaminophen overdose
Special Considerations	Can also be used for some bronchial diseases

Drug Class	Muscle Relaxants
Indication	To reduce muscle tension
Examples	• baclofen (Lioresal®) • carisoprodol (Soma®) • cyclobenzaprine (Flexeril®)
Special Considerations	Carisoprodol (Soma®) is a schedule IV controlled substance

Drug Class	Disease-Modifying Antirheumatic Agents (DMARDs)
Indication	To treat rheumatoid arthritis
Examples	• abatacept (Orencia®) • adalimumab (Humira®) • etanercept (Enbrel®) • methotrexate (Rheumatrex®)
Special Considerations	Helps slow the progression of the disease, but use is limited by side effects

ANTIEPILEPTIC/ANTICONVULSANT

. . . .

ANTI-PARKINSON'S AGENTS

. . . .

ANTI-ALZHEIMER'S DISEASE AGENTS

Drug Class	Antiepileptic/Anticonvulsant
Description of Condition	Epilepsy is a disorder characterized by recurrent seizures.
Indication	Used to treat epilepsy
Examples of Antiepileptic/ Anticonvulsant Agents	• carbamazepine (Tegretol®) • clonazepam (Klonopin®) • divalproex (Depakote®) • lamotrigine (Lamictal®) • levetiracetam (Keppra®) • pregabalin (Lyrica®) • topiramate (Topamax®) • phenytoin sodium (Dilantin®)
Special Considerations	Can cause sedation and loss of cognition, so poor compliance is an issue; large number of drug interactions can occur

. . . .

Drug Class	Anti-Parkinson's Agents
Description of Condition	Parkinson's disease is characterized by muscular difficulties, including tremors and loss of muscle control; generally affects patients over age 60
Indication	Used to treat symptoms of Parkinson's disease
Examples of Anti-Parkinson's Agents	• levodopa-carbidopa (Sinemet®) • amantadine (Symmetrel®) • benztropine (Cogentin®) • ropinirole (Requip®)
Special Considerations	Side effects are a problem and sometimes require constant change in medication.

. . . .

Drug Class	Anti-Alzheimer's Disease Agents
Description of Condition	Alzheimer's disease is a neurodegenerative disease that leads to dementia.
Indication	Used to treat symptoms of Alzheimer's disease
Examples of Anti-Alzheimer's Disease Agents	• donepezil (Aricept®) • gingko • memantine (Namenda®) • rivastigmine (Exelon®)
Special Considerations	Drugs can slow disease, but not cure or reverse effects

ADD/ADHD AGENTS

....

ANTIASTHMATICS

....

BRONCHODILATORS

Drug Class	ADD/ADHD Agents
Description of Condition	Attention deficit disorder (ADD) and attention deficit hyperactivity disorder (ADHD) are characterized by hyperactivity and distractibility.
Indication	Used to treat attention disorders such as ADD/ADHD
Examples of ADD/ADHD Agents	**Stimulants** • amphetamine with dextroamphetamine salts (Adderall®) • methylphenidate (Concerta®, Ritalin®, Metadate CD®) **Nonstimulants** • atomoxetine (Straterra®) • guanfacine (Intuniv®)
Special Considerations	Stimulants are schedule II controlled substances because of their amphetamine derivative.

Drug Class	Antiasthmatics
Description of Condition	Asthma is an inflammatory condition of the lungs that causes airway constriction; characterized by wheezing, coughing, and difficulty breathing
Indication	Used to treat asthma and breathing disorders
Drug Classes	• bronchodilators • corticosteroids • leukotriene inhibitors • mast cell stabilizers • xanthine derivatives

Drug Class	Bronchodilators
Mechanism of Action	Relaxes smooth muscle cells of the bronchioles, resulting in an increase in airway diameter
Indication	Used to treat asthma, COPD, and chronic bronchitis
Examples	• albuterol (Proventil HFA®, Proair HFA®, Ventolin HFA®) • ipratropium (Atrovent®) • salmeterol (Serevent®) • tiotropium (Spiriva®)

CORTICOSTEROIDS

. . . .

LEUKOTRIENE INHIBITORS

. . . .

MAST CELL STABILIZERS

Drug Class	Corticosteroids
Mechanism of Action	Inhibit the immune system to suppress inflammation
Indication	Used to treat inflammatory conditions, and suppresses the immune response
Examples	• prednisone (Deltasone®) • prednisolone (Orapred®) • methylprednisolone (Medrol®) • triamcinolone (Azmacort®) • fluticasone (Flovent®, Flonase®) • fluticasone and salmeterol (Advair®)
Special Considerations	**Inhaled corticosteroids** • patients must rinse mouth after use to prevent thrush **Oral corticosteroids** • long-term use can cause weight gain, buffalo hump, and moon face or facial hair in females, and breast development in males

Drug Class	Leukotriene Inhibitors
Mechanism of Action	Block leukotrienes, which results in the blocking of inflammatory responses
Indication	Used for prophylactic treatment of asthma
Example	• montelukast (Singulair®)
Special Considerations	Singulair® can be used in patients as young as 12 months old

Drug Class	Mast Cell Stabilizers
Mechanism of Action	Inhibit inflammatory cells
Indication	Used for prophylactic treatment of asthma
Examples	• cromolyn (Intal®, NasalCrom®) • nedocromil (Tilade®)
Special Considerations	A bronchodilator is used first so that airways are opened prior to use, which may cause poor compliance; also has unpleasant taste and can cause hoarseness and dry mouth

XANTHINE DERIVATIVES

....

SMOKING CESSATION AGENTS

....

TUBERCULOSIS AGENTS

Drug Class	Xanthine Derivatives
Mechanism of Action	Relax airway smooth muscle, leading to opening of airways and increased air movement
Indication	Used for treatment of lung diseases unresponsive to other treatments
Examples	• aminophylline • theophylline
Special Considerations	Theophylline has many interactions and is used only if asthma or other lung disease is unresponsive to other treatments.

Drug Class	Smoking Cessation Agents
Description of Condition	Smoking can increase risk of cancer, COPD, heart disease, and stroke
Examples	• buproprion (Wellbutrin®, Zyban®) • nicotine (Nicoderm®, Nicotrol®, Nicorette®) • varenicline (Chantix®)

Drug Class	Tuberculosis Agents
Description of Condition	Disease of the respiratory tract caused by a bacteria; patients have a long drug therapy consisting of many medications, which leads to poor compliance
Indication	Used for treatment of tuberculosis
Examples	• isoniazid (INH) • rifampin (Rifadin®) • ethambutol (Myambutol®)
Special Considerations	• Patients should avoid alcohol with all drugs. • Rifampin causes discoloration of urine, tears, sweat and any body fluids—turns all fluids a reddish orange

ANTACIDS

. . . .

H$_2$ RECEPTOR BLOCKERS

. . . .

PROTON PUMP INHIBITORS

Drug Class	Antacids
Mechanism of Action	Neutralize stomach acid
Indication	Used for treatment of gastroesophageal reflux disease (GERD) and heartburn
Examples	• aluminum hydroxide-magnesium hydroxide-simethicone (Mylanta®, Maalox®) • magnesium hydroxide (Milk of Magnesia®) • calcium carbonate (Tums®)
Special Considerations	Available OTC

. . . .

Drug Class	H₂ Receptor Blockers
Mechanism of Action	Block gastric acid and secretion from histamine through blockage at the H_2 receptor
Indication	Used for treatment of gastroesophageal reflux disease (GERD) and heartburn
Examples	• cimetidine (Tagamet®) • nizatidine (Axid®) • ranitidine (Zantac®) • famotidine (Pepcid®)
Special Considerations	All are available OTC; important to take at bedtime
Hint	-tidine ending for H₂ Receptor Blockers

. . . .

Drug Class	Proton Pump Inhibitors
Mechanism of Action	Block the proton pump, which normally pumps acidic ions into the stomach—this reduces stomach acidity
Indication	Used for treatment of gastroesophageal reflux disease (GERD) and heartburn; can also be used in ulcer therapy
Examples	• esomeprazole (Nexium®) • lansoprazole (Prevacid®) • omeprazole (Prilosec®) • pantoprazole (Protonix®)
Special Considerations	Must be taken on a daily basis for effectiveness
Hint	-prazole ending for Proton Pump Inhibitors (PPIs)

ANTIDIARRHEALS

. . . .

LAXATIVES

. . . .

BULK-FORMING LAXATIVES

Drug Class	Antidiarrheals
Mechanism of Action	Decrease bowel motility and act as a water adsorbent
Indication	Used for symptomatic relief of diarrhea
Examples	• diphenoxylate with atropine (Lomotil® C-V) • loperamide (Imodium®) • bismuth subsalicylate (Pepto Bismol®)
Special Considerations	Diarrhea can lead to dehydration and should be monitored.

. . . .

Drug Class	Laxatives
Description of Condition	Constipation is the difficulty or inability to pass bowel movements.
Indication	Used for treatment of constipation
Types of Laxatives	• bulk-forming • saline • stimulant • stool softeners • bowel evacuants

. . . .

Drug Class	Bulk-Forming Laxatives
Mechanism of Action	Increase stool size, which promotes intestinal movement and bowel movement
Indication	Used for the treatment of constipation
Examples	• psyllium hydrophilic mucilloid (Metamucil®)
Special Considerations	Patient must drink plenty of water to avoid further constipation, can be taken on a daily basis

SALINE LAXATIVES

. . . .

STIMULANT LAXATIVES

. . . .

STOOL SOFTENERS

Drug Class	Saline Laxatives
Mechanism of Action	Draw water into the colon to promote bowel evacuation
Indication	Used for the treatment of constipation
Examples	• lactulose (Enulose®) • magnesium hydroxide (Milk of Magnesia®) • sodium phosphate (Fleet Phospho-Soda®)
Special Considerations	Patient must drink plenty of water to avoid further constipation

. . . .

Drug Class	Stimulant Laxatives
Mechanism of Action	Stimulate the gut through irritation of the lining, which increases contractions and bowel movements
Indication	Used for the treatment of constipation
Examples	• bisacodyl (Dulcolax®) • senna (Senokot®)
Special Considerations	Be careful of overuse—can cause the bowel to become dependent on laxative use

. . . .

Drug Class	Stool Softeners
Mechanism of Action	Allow fluids to mix into the bowel and stool, which creates a softer and easier-to-pass stool
Indication	Used for the treatment of constipation
Example	• docusate (Colace®)

Pharmacology—Drug Classes

BOWEL EVACUANT LAXATIVES

. . . .

ANTIEMETICS

. . . .

WEIGHT-LOSS MEDICATIONS

[111]

PHARMACY TECHNICIAN FLASH REVIEW

Drug Class	Bowel Evacuant Laxatives
Mechanism of Action	Draw a large amount of water into the bowels, which creates watery stools
Indication	Used for the treatment of nausea
Example	• polyethylene glycol-electrolyte solution (GoLYTELY®)
Special Considerations	Eight ounces is taken every 10 minutes until 4 liters can be consumed; food should not be eaten at least 3 hours prior to administration

· ·

Drug Class	Antiemetics
Mechanism of Action	Inhibit the impulse that goes from the chemoreceptor trigger zone (CTZ), or part of the brain that induces vomiting to the stomach
Indication	Used for the treatment of nausea
Examples	• metoclopramide (Reglan®) • ondansetron (Zofran®) • promethazine (Phenergan®)
Side Effects	Dizziness, drowsiness

· ·

Drug Class	Weight-Loss Medications
Indication	Used for the treatment of obesity
Examples	• orlistat (Xenical®) • phentermine (Ionamin®) • siburtramine (Meridia®)
Special Considerations	Some are stimulants and controlled substances

DIURETICS

. . . .

LOOP DIURETICS

. . . .

THIAZIDE DIURETICS

Drug Class	Diuretics
Indication	Used to maintain the balance of water, electrolytes, and acids and bases
Types of Diuretics	• loop • potassium sparing • thiazides • combination
Special Considerations	Diuretics should be avoided at bedtime to prevent frequent urination at night

- -

Drug Class	Loop Diuretics
Mechanism of Action	Inhibit the reabsorption of sodium and chloride in the loop of Henle, which results in excretion of water
Indication	Used for the treatment of hypertension, edema, and congestive heart failure (CHF)
Examples	• furosemide (Lasix®) • bumetanide (Bumex®) • torsemide (Demadex®)

- -

Drug Class	Thiazide Diuretics
Mechanism of Action	Inhibit reabsorption of sodium and chloride ions in the distal convoluted tubule of the kidney, which promotes water excretion
Indication	Used for the treatment of hypertension, edema, and congestive heart failure (CHF)
Example	• hydrochlorothiazide (Hydrodiuril®)
Special Considerations	May cause hypokalemia (low potassium)

POTASSIUM-SPARING DIURETICS

. . . .

ALPHA BLOCKERS

. . . .

ANTIHYPERTENSIVES

Drug Class	Potassium-Sparing Diuretics
Mechanism of Action	Block sodium and potassium exchange at the distal convoluted tubule, or competitively inhibit aldosterone
Indication	Used for adjunctive treatment of hypertension and edema
Examples	• spironolactone (Aldactone®) • triamterene (Dyrenium®)
Special Considerations	Should be avoided in patients taking ACE inhibitors (both have potassium-sparing effect and can cause hyperkalemia—excessive potassium in the blood)
Combination Diuretics	Triamterene can be given with hydrochlorothiazide for an added effect • triamterene with hydrochlorothiazide—tablet (Maxzide®) • triamterene with hydrochlorothiazide—capsule (Dyazide®)

Drug Class	Alpha Blockers
Mechanism of Action	Block peripheral alpha receptors, which relaxes smooth muscle, especially in the prostate—this helps reduce urinary symptoms associated with benign prostatic hyperplasia (BPH)
Indication	Used for the treatment of prostate disease
Examples	• alfuzosin (Uroxatral®) • doxazosin (Cardura®) • dutasteride (Avodart®) • tamsulosin (Flomax®) • terazosin (Hytrin®)

Drug Class	Antihypertensives
Description of Condition	Hypertension is high blood pressure, which consists of pressure at least 140/90 mmHg or higher on a consistent basis
Indication	Used for the treatment of hypertension
Types of Antihypertensives	• diuretics • angiotensin-converting enzyme (ACE) inhibitors • angiotensin-II receptor blockers (ARBs) • beta blockers • calcium channel blockers • combination products

PHARMACY TECHNICIAN FLASH REVIEW

ANGIOTENSIN CONVERTING ENZYME (ACE) INHIBITORS

. . . .

ANGIOTENSIN II RECEPTOR BLOCKERS (ARBs)

. . . .

BETA BLOCKERS

Drug Class	Angiotensin Converting Enzyme (ACE) Inhibitors
Mechanism of Action	Block angiotensin converting enzyme (ACE), which prevents the conversion of angiotensin I to angiotensin II, and thus reduces vasoconstriction and blood pressure (see picture)
Indication	Used for the treatment of hypertension
Examples	• benazepril (Lotensin®) • enalapril (Vasotec®) • lisinopril (Prinivil®, Zestril®) • quinapril (Accupril®) • ramipril (Altace®)
Special Considerations	Should be avoided in patients taking potassium-sparing diuretics
Hint	-pril ending for generic ACE inhibitors

```
Angiotensin I
    ⇓
Angiotensin II        ACE Inhibitors
    ⇓
Angiotensin II Receptors
    ⇓
Vasoconstriction
```

Drug Class	Angiotensin II Receptor Blockers (ARBs)
Mechanism of Action	Block angiotensin II receptors and vasoconstriction from occurring, thus lowering blood pressure (see picture)
Indication	Used for the treatment of hypertension
Examples	• irbesartan (Avapro®) • losartan (Cozaar®) • olmesartan (Benicar®) • valsartan (Diovan®)
Hint	-sartan ending for generic ARBs

```
Angiotensin I
    ⇓
Angiotensin II        ACE
    ⇓
ARBs
```

Drug Class	Beta Blockers
Mechanism of Action	Block beta receptors, which decreases heart rate and lowers blood pressure
Indication	Used for the treatment of hypertension
Examples	• atenolol (Tenormin®) • carvedilol (Coreg®) • propranolol (Inderal®)
Hint	-lol ending for generic beta blockers
Special Considerations	Contraindicated in patients with asthma

PHARMACY TECHNICIAN FLASH REVIEW

CALCIUM CHANNEL BLOCKERS

. . . .

ANTIARRHYTHMICS

. . . .

ANTIANGINAL AGENTS

Drug Class	Calcium Channel Blockers
Mechanism of Action	Inhibit calcium ions from entering channels of the heart muscle, resulting in relaxation of smooth muscle and vasodilation
Indication	Used for the treatment of hypertension
Examples	• amlodipine (Norvasc®) • diltiazem (Cardizem®) • nifedipine (Procardia®) • verapamil (Calan®, Isoptin®)

Drug Class	Antiarrhythmics
Description of Condition	Arrhythmias result when the ventricular and atrial contractions are not synchronized; can include tachycardia, atrial flutter, and fibrillation
Indication	Used for the treatment of arrhythmias
Types of Antiarrhythmics	• channel blockers • membrane-stabilizing agents • potassium channel blockers

Drug Class	Antianginal Agents
Description of Condition	Angina is a disease marked by severe chest pain due to an insufficient amount of blood carrying oxygen.
Indication	Used for the treatment of angina
Types of Antianginal Agents	• beta blockers • calcium channel blockers • nitrates
Special Considerations	Treatment aimed at reducing angina attacks and preventing a heart attack.

NITRATES

. . . .

ANTICOAGULANT

. . . .

ANTIPLATELET

Drug Class	Nitrates
Mechanism of Action	Relax the smooth muscle of the heart and dilate the surrounding blood vessels to increase blood flow
Indication	Used for the treatment of angina
Examples	• isosorbide dinitrate (Isordil®) • isosorbide mononitrate (Imdur®) • nitroglycerin (Nitrquick®, Nitrostat®)
Special Considerations	Nitroglycerin is used sublingually as the drug of choice for an acute attack of angina; nitrates should not be used if taking specific medications for erectile dysfunction—can cause an unsafe drop in blood pressure

Drug Class	Anticoagulant
Mechanism of Action	Prevent the formation of clots by inhibiting clotting factors in the blood
Indication	Used for the prevention of blood clots
Examples	• heparin (not available orally) • warfarin (Coumadin®)
Special Considerations	Patients should avoid foods with Vitamin K when taking warfarin; heparin is always given via IV or subcutaneously; patients must always be monitored while on anticoagulant therapy
Remember	Anticoagulant drugs cannot dissolve clots that are already present, but only prevent others from occurring.

Drug Class	Antiplatelet
Mechanism of Action	Interfere with reactions that cause platelets to clot
Indication	Used for the prevention of blood clots
Examples	• aspirin • clopidogrel (Plavix®)
Special Considerations	Patients should not start aspirin therapy without first consulting their doctors.
Remember	Antiplatelet drugs cannot dissolve clots that are already present, but only prevent others from occurring.

FIBRINOLYTICS

. . . .

ANTIHYPERLIPIDEMICS

. . . .

HMG-CoA REDUCTASE INHIBITORS

Drug Class	Fibrinolytics
Mechanism of Action	Dissolve clots by binding to clotting agent and preventing it from holding the clot together
Indication	Used to dissolve preexisting blood clots
Examples	• alteplase (Activase®) • reteplase (Retavase®) • renecteplase (TNKase®)
Special Considerations	All fibrinolytics are in powder form and must be reconstituted.
Remember	Fibrinolytics are the only type of drug that can dissolve a preexisting clot.

Drug Class	Antihyperlipidemics
Description of Condition	Elevation of cholesterol levels; above 240 mg per 100 mL of blood is "at risk"
Indication	Used for the treatment of high cholesterol
Types of Antihyperlipidemics	• bile acid sequestrants • fibric acid derivatives • HMG-CoA reductase inhibitors • combination drugs

Drug Class	HMG-CoA Reductase Inhibitors
Mechanism of Action	Inhibit the enzyme that is required for cholesterol production
Indication	Used to lower cholesterol
Examples	• atorvastatin (Lipitor®) • lovastatin (Mevacor®) • pravastatin (Pravachol®) • rosuvastatin (Crestor®) • simvastatin (Zocor®)
Special Considerations	Most work better when taken at night; patients should avoid drinking grapefruit juice
Hint	Also known as "statins" because generics end in –statin

HYPOTHYROIDISM

. . . .

HYPERTHYROIDISM

. . . .

HORMONE REPLACEMENT THERAPY

Drug Class	Hypothyroidism
Description of Condition	Underactive thyroid, which produces insufficient amounts of thyroid hormones; characterized by weight gain and decreased heart rate in adults
Treated with	Thyroid replacement therapy
Examples	• levothyroxine (Levothroid®, Levoxyl®, Synthroid®) • thyroid (Armour Thyroid®)

. . . .

Drug Class	Hyperthyroidism
Description of Condition	Overactive thyroid, which produces excessive amounts of thyroid hormones; may be caused by a tumor or excessive iodine intake
Treated with	Surgery or drug treatment
Examples	• methimazole (Tapazole®) • propylthiouracil (PTU®) • radioactive iodine ^{131}I

. . . .

Drug Class	Hormone Replacement Therapy
Description of Condition	Treatment helps relieve symptoms of estrogen deficiency resulting from menopause
Symptoms	• severe hot flashes • vaginal atrophy • insomnia • irritability
Examples	• conjugated estrogen (Premarin®) • conjugated estrogen-medroxyprogesterone (Prempro®, Premphase®, estradiol-levonorgestrel (Climara®)

ORAL CONTRACEPTIVES

. . . .

OSTEOPOROSIS AGENTS

. . . .

BISPHOSPHONATES

Drug Class	Oral Contraceptives
Mechanism of Action	Suppress ovulation by interfering with hormone production
Indication	Used to prevent pregnancy
Examples	• ethinyl estradiol with levonorgestrel (Triphasil®) • ethinyl estradiol with norgestimate (Ortho Tri-Cyclen®) • ethinyl estradiol with norgestrel (Lo-Ovral®) • ethinyl estradiol with drospirinone (Yasmin®)
Special Considerations	Most are a combination of estrogen (ethinyl estradiol) and progesterone
Emergency Contraceptive	Levonorgestrel (Plan B®) available OTC

Drug Class	Osteoporosis Agents
Description of Condition	Decreased bone density resulting from a deficiency in estrogen, calcium, and/or vitamin D
Examples of Osteoporosis Agents	• bisphosphonates • OTC calcium • calcitonin-salmon (Miacalcin®) nasal spray • raloxifene (Evista®)

Drug Class	Bisphosphonates
Mechanism of Action	Prevent the bone from being reabsorbed and broken down by osteoclasts
Indication	Used to treat osteoporosis
Examples	• alendronate (Fosamax®) • ibandronate (Boniva®) • risedronate (Actonel®)
Special Considerations	Should be taken before the first meal of the day and with six to eight ounces of water—patient must also remain upright for at least half an hour after taking to prevent heartburn
Hint	-dronate ending for generic bisphosphonates

PHARMACY TECHNICIAN FLASH REVIEW

ANTIDIABETICS

. . . .

INSULIN

. . . .

ORAL HYPOGLYCEMIC AGENTS

Drug Class	Antidiabetics
Description of Condition	Type 1 diabetes • patient is unable to produce any insulin, requires insulin therapy Type 2 diabetes • patient's body does not respond to insulin secretion, or has impaired insulin secretion Gestational diabetes • results from pregnancy Secondary diabetes • results from another medication
Treatment Methods	Depends on type of diabetes; can be treated with insulin or oral hypoglycemic medications

Drug Class	Insulin
Mechanism of Action	Lowers blood sugar in patients who are unable to make insulin
Indication	Used to treat diabetes
Examples	**Rapid** • lispro (Humalog®), aspart (Novolog®), regular (Humulin-R®, Novolin-R®) **Intermediate** • Humulin N, Humulin 70/30 **Long** • detemir (Levemir®), glargine (Lantus®)
Special Considerations	Must be given subcutaneously; injection site should be rotated

Drug Class	Oral Hypoglycemic Agents
Mechanism of Action	Improve response to insulin and glucose
Indication	Used to treat non-insulin dependent diabetes
Examples	• glimepiride (Amaryl®) • glipizide (Glucotrol®) • glyburide (DiaBeta®, Micronase®) • metformin (Glucophage®) • pioglitazone (Actos®)
Special Considerations	Because they improve the response of the body to insulin, and Type I diabetics do not produce insulin, these drugs are not indicated for Type I diabetes; changing of diet and increasing exercise (lifestyle change) should also be included in therapy.

ANTINEOPLASTICS

. . . .

GLAUCOMA AGENTS

. . . .

ANTI-ACNE AGENTS

Drug Class	Antineoplastics
Description of Condition	Cancer is a disease of uncontrolled abnormal cellular growth.
Indication	Used for the treatment of cancer
Examples of Antineoplastics	• alkylating agents • antibiotics • antimetabolites • hormones • nitrogen mustards • plant alkaloids
Special Considerations	Chemotherapy drugs must never be handled by technicians who are pregnant.

. . . .

Drug Class	Glaucoma Agents
Description of Condition	Glaucoma is a disorder of the eye characterized by intraocular pressure that can destroy nerves and lead to vision loss.
Mechanism of Action	Lower pressure by increasing drainage or decreasing production of aqueous humor
Indication	Used for the treatment of glaucoma
Examples of Glaucoma Agents	• bimatoprost (Lumigan®) • brimonidine (Alphagan P®) • dorzolaminde (Trusopt®) • latanoprost (Xalatan®) • timolol (Timoptic®)

. . . .

Drug Class	Anti-Acne Agents
Description of Condition	Acne vulgaris generally starts at puberty due to an increase in sebum secretion from sebaceous glands.
Indication	Used for the treatment of acne
Examples of Glaucoma Agents	• adapalene (Differin®) • clindamycin with benzyl peroxide (BenzaClin®) • isotretinoin (Accutain®)
Special Considerations	Products can come in many different dosage forms; isotretinoin patients must participate in the iPLEDGE program, which requires females to undergo pregnancy testing and be on oral contraceptives prior to use.

VITAMIN

. . . .

FAT SOLUBLE VITAMINS

. . . .

WATER SOLUBLE VITAMINS

Essential organic compounds required by an organism in a limited amount for necessary functions.

May be either:

Fat soluble: excessive intake can result in toxicity, as these vitamins can accumulate and are stored in the body – Vitamins A, D, E, and K

Water soluble: eliminated by the kidneys, so overdosing is less likely to be as dangerous as a fat-soluble overdose – Vitamins B Complex and C

. . . .

Fat soluble vitamins

Vitamin	Generic Name	Function in the Body
A	Retinol	Bone health and growth, eyes (retina function), and reproduction
D	Ergocalciferol	Bone health
E	Tocopherol	Antioxidant and enhances immune response
K	Phytonadione	Blood clotting

. . . .

Water soluble vitamins

Vitamin	Generic Name	Function in the Body
B_1	Thiamine	Important for energy production and heart and muscle function
B_2	Riboflavin	Important for energy production and hair, skin, and nails
B_3	Nicotinic Acid	Involved in fat synthesis and protein metabolism, also called **niacin**
B_5	Pantothenic Acid	Important for energy and normal growth
B_6	Pyridoxine	Helps in metabolism and red blood cell production
B_7	Biotin	Necessary for cell growth, may strengthen nails
B_9	Folic Acid	Essential for healthy fetal development in pregnant women
B_{12}	Cyanocobalamin	Important for red blood cell production
C	Ascorbic Acid	Helps in the immune process and promotes healing

ERECTILE DYSFUNCTION (ED) MEDICATIONS

. . . .

ALTERNATIVE SUPPLEMENTS

. . . .

Drug Class	Erectile Dysfunction (ED) Medications
Description of Condition	Occurs when a man cannot keep an erection long enough or firm enough for sexual intercourse
Indication	Used for the treatment of ED
Examples of ED Agents	Phosphodiesterase Inhibitors • sildenafil (Viagra®) • tadalafil (Cialis®) • vardenafil (Levitra®, Staxyn®)
Special Considerations	These products should never be used in patients taking nitrates for chest pain—can cause an unsafe drop in blood pressure

Alternative Supplement	Common Use
Chondroitin	Osteoarthritis
Cranberry	Urinary health
Echinacea	Colds
Evening primrose	Premenstrual symptoms
Fish oil	Blood pressure and cholesterol
Garlic	Cholesterol and cardiovascular health
Ginger	Nausea, GI upset
Ginkgo biloba	Improve memory and prevent dementia
Ginseng	Fatigue
Glucosamine	Osteoarthritis
Grape seed	Allergies
Green tea	Metabolic syndromes
Kava kava	Stress and anxiety, sedative effects
Melatonin	Insomnia, jet lag
Milk thistle	Liver disease
St. John's Wort	Depression
Saw palmetto	Prostate disorders
Soy	Menopausal symptoms
Valerian	Anxiety

MINERALS

．．．

Mineral	Chemical Symbol	Use in the Body
Calcium	Ca	Nerve and muscle function, bone and tooth formation
Copper	Cu	Blood formation
Iodine	I	Thyroid function
Iron	Fe	Red blood cell formation
Magnesium	Mg	Muscle function
Potassium	K	Heart and nerve function, cellular balance
Sodium	Na	Nerve and muscle function, cellular balance
Sulfur	S	Energy production and cellular function
Zinc	Zn	Immunity

ADVERSE DRUG REACTION (ADR)

. . . .

THERAPEUTIC EQUIVALENCE

. . . .

THERAPEUTIC EQUIVALENCY CODES

. . . .

ORANGE BOOK

When a patient receives a medication at a normal dosage range but experiences a harmful reaction as a result of the medication.

. . . .

When two drugs can be substituted and have the same affect both clinically and in safety profiles; they must be the same dosage form, strength, route of administration, and contain the same active ingredient.

. . . .

Also known as TE codes; coding process the FDA uses to determine whether a product is therapeutically equivalent.

- A drug is given a rating of **A** if the FDA can demonstrate through studies that it is therapeutically equivalent.

- A drug is given a rating of **B** if it is not therapeutically equivalent.

. . . .

An online resource published by the FDA that provides information on therapeutic equivalencies and TE Codes.

DRUG INTERACTION

. . . .

DRUG-DRUG INTERACTION

. . . .

DRUG-DISEASE INTERACTION

When a drug interacts with another substance when taken concurrently.

. . . .

The interaction of two drugs when taken together that differs in the response that would occur if each were taken alone; can usually be classified as one of the following types of interactions:

• Synergy—when two drugs taken together have a more intense effect than when each would be taken separately

• Antagonism—when two drugs are taken together, and one drug negates the effect of the other drug

. . . .

An effect a drug has on the disease state or pathological condition of a patient; can be either a positive or negative effect.

DRUG-FOOD INTERACTION

. . . .

DRUG

. . . .

ACTIVE INGREDIENT

When the effect of a drug is altered due to the consumption of a particular food or drink; this could prevent the drug from working, enhance or decrease side effects, or cause the development of a new side effect.

. . . .

A substance that alters the body in a specific way and is used in the treatment, prevention, or diagnosis of a disease.

Can be:

• Therapeutic—relieves symptoms of a disease

• Prophylactic—prevents or decreases severity of a disease

Names of drugs:

• Chemical Name—describes the chemical makeup of a drug

• Generic Name—name given to drug that is not protected by a trademark, also known as the United States Adopted Name (USAN)

• Brand/Trade Name—name by which the manufacturer markets the drug, is protected by a trademark

. . . .

The part of the drug that alters the body to produce the desired effect.

INACTIVE INGREDIENT

....

PLACEBO

....

DOSAGE FORM

Has no effect on the therapeutic action of a drug; also known as excipient or inert ingredients.

Examples:

- colorings

- flavorings

- preservatives

- fillers

. . . .

A substance that has no medicinal treatment value, often used in medical research for studies.

. . . .

The physical form the drug is dispensed as.

Example: tablet, capsule, liquid

PRODUCT PACKAGE INSERT (PPI)

. . . .

BLACK BOX WARNING

. . . .

Information sent from the wholesaler on a medication for the pharmacy to utilize for any material needed regarding a specific drug; written for the pharmacist and technician—not for the patient.

. . . .

A warning communicated to medical personnel through product package inserts that alerts physicians to serious adverse reaction potential of specific medications.

Example:

HIGHLIGHTS OF PRESCRIBING INFORMATION
These highlights do not include all the information needed to use LEVAQUIN® safely and effectively. See full prescribing information for LEVAQUIN®.

LEVAQUIN® (levofloxacin) Tablets
LEVAQUIN® (levofloxacin) Oral Solution
LEVAQUIN® (levofloxacin) Injection, for Intravenous Use
LEVAQUIN® (levofloxacin in 5% dextrose) Injection, for Intravenous Use
Initial U.S. Approval: 1996

WARNING:
Fluoroquinolones, including LEVAQUIN®, are associated with an increased risk of tendinitis and tendon rupture in all ages. This risk is further increased in older patients usually over 60 years of age, in patients taking corticosteroid drugs, and in patients with kidney, heart or lung transplants [See *Warnings and Precautions (5.1)*].

. . . .

HALF-LIFE

· ·

ADME

· ·

The amount of time it takes the body to eliminate half of a specific drug.

Example: The half-life of a drug is 5 hours, and the original dose is 20 mg—it will take 15 hours for this drug to be eliminated down to 2.5 mg:

$$20/2 = 10 \text{ mg over 5 hours}$$

$$10/2 = 5 \text{ mg over 5 hours}$$

$$\underline{5/2 = 2.5 \text{ mg over 5 hours}}$$

15 hours total to eliminate the drug down to 2.5 mg

· ·

Absorption—the process of a drug entering the bloodstream

Distribution—the process of a drug moving from the blood into the tissues and cells to elicit the action of the drug

Metabolism—the process of a drug being converted to a form that is easily eliminated from the body

Excretion/Elimination—the process of removing a drug from the body, usually through urine (kidneys)

· ·

ORAL SYRINGE

. . . .

SUBLINGUAL

. . . .

BUCCAL

PHARMACY TECHNICIAN FLASH REVIEW

A syringe used to measure liquids to be given orally to pediatric patients. Comes with a cap so that doses can be dispensed for individual patients.

· ·

A method of drug delivery that involves placing a tablet under the tongue to be dissolved; the tablet can be absorbed quickly into the bloodstream through the blood vessels under the tongue.

- A common sublingual medication is nitroglycerin, used for angina attacks.

· ·

A method of drug delivery in which a medication is placed into the cheek pouch and absorbed through the blood vessels of the cheek.

OPHTHALMIC

. . . .

OTIC

. . . .

NASAL

Application of a drug into the eye; **must be a sterile solution**.

. . . .

Application of a drug into the ear; medications used for the ear **can never be used in the eye**; however, if necessary **eye drops can be used in the ear**.

. . . .

Application of a drug into the nose; most often given in spray form.

SUPPOSITORY

. . . .

ENEMA

. . . .

VAGINAL

A dosage form in a semi-solid state that is solid at room temperature but designed to melt at body temperature; usually inserted rectally, can also be inserted vaginally or into the urethra.

· ·

A solution that is administered rectally for bowel cleansing and evacuation; given prior to a procedure or for a specific treatment.

· ·

Application of a drug into the vagina; used mostly for local effects such as the treatment of yeast infections.

RECTAL

. . . .

URETHRAL

. . . .

TOPICAL

Administration of a drug into the rectum; usually given via suppositories, but also may be given through an enema.

· ·

Administration of a drug through the urethra, the tube that carries the urine from the bladder to the outside of the body; usually used for cancer or incontinence treatment.

· ·

Any medication that is applied directly to the surface of the skin for localized effects.

INHALATION

. . . .

METERED-DOSE INHALER (MDI)

. . . .

NEBULIZER

Administration of a drug through inhalation into the lungs, used mostly for asthma and COPD treatment methods.

· ·

Propellant inhaler used by asthma patients that delivers a specific amount of medication through compressed gas.

· ·

A machine used for administering medication into the lungs of children or other patients requiring a breathing treatment; patient will wear a mask, and the medication is delivered as a fine mist that the patient breathes in to make sure it reaches the lungs.

SPACER

. . . .

PARENTERAL

. . . .

INTRAVENOUS

A tubelike attachment to an MDI inhaler that helps patients, typically children, inhale the medication more easily and effectively.

. . . .

Administration of a drug that involves any type of injection that bypasses the stomach; because it enters the bloodstream directly, it must be a sterile dosage form.

. . . .

Also known as IV, administration of a drug directly into the bloodstream through a vein.

Examples of medications given intravenously:

- antibiotics

- analgesics

- anticoagulants such as heparin

IV BOLUS

. . . .

IV INFUSION

. . . .

LOADING DOSE

PHARMACY TECHNICIAN FLASH REVIEW

Used when rapid administration of a drug is required; medication is pushed all at once, such as when patients receive epinephrine during cardiac arrest; also known as IV push.

· ·

Used to provide administration of an intravenous drug over a longer period of time; medication is hung in bags, and the infusion rate is calculated to determine the quantity needed for the entire duration of therapy.

· ·

A larger dose of a medication given to a patient to bring the concentration of drug in the blood to a therapeutic level more rapidly than a single dose; maintained at therapeutic level with a maintenance dose.

PHARMACY TECHNICIAN FLASH REVIEW

IV PIGGYBACK

. . . .

INTRAMUSCULAR

. . . .

SUBCUTANEOUS

. . . .

INTRADERMAL

PHARMACY TECHNICIAN FLASH REVIEW

Used for administration of an intravenous medication using the primary IV line already being used for IV infusion; a second bag is hung with the medication needed to be infused simultaneously as the main infusion.

. . . .

Administration of medication injected into the muscle; typically no more than 2 mL of liquid can be injected, but can go up to 5 mL; common injection sites are gluteus maximus (butt) and deltoid (shoulder); inject at 90-degree angle.

. . . .

Administration of medication directly below the skin into the subcutaneous tissue; example of a medication administered via this route is insulin; inject at a 45-degree angle.

. . . .

Administration of medication given just below the epidermis (top layer of the skin); must only inject a small amount of medication—will raise the skin to form a wheal. Example: tuberculosis skin tests are administered intradermally.

HYDROCODONE WITH ACETAMINOPHEN

. . . .

LISINOPRIL

. . . .

LEVOTHYROXINE SODIUM

Generic Name	**Hydrocodone with Acetaminophen**
Brand Name	Lorcet®, Lortab®, Norco®, Vicodin®
Drug Class	Opioid analgesic
Indication	Relief of moderate to moderately severe pain
Controlled Substance	C-III

. . . .

Generic Name	**Lisinipril**
Brand Name	Prinivil®, Zestril®
Drug Class	Antihypertensive: ACE inhibitor
Indication	Treatment of high blood pressure (hypertension)
Hint	ACE Inhibitor generic names end in *-pril*

. . . .

Generic Name	**Levothyroxine**
Brand Name	Levoxyl®, Synthroid®, Unithroid®, Levothroid®
Drug Class	Thyroid hormone
Indication	Treatment of hypothyroidism

SIMVASTATIN

. . . .

OMEPRAZOLE

. . . .

METFORMIN HYDROCHLORIDE

PHARMACY TECHNICIAN FLASH REVIEW

Generic Name	Simvastatin
Brand Name	Zocor®
Drug Class	Antihyperlipidemic—HMG-CoA Reductase Inhibitor (statin)
Indication	Treatment of high cholesterol
Hint	-statin ending for HMG-CoA Reductase Inhibitors for high cholesterol

Generic Name	Omeprazole
Brand Name	Prilosec®
Drug Class	Antiulcer agent—Proton Pump Inhibitor (PPI)
Indication	Treatment of Gastroesophageal Reflux Disease (GERD), ulcers, acid reflux, and other hypersecretory conditions
Hint	-prazole generic ending for Proton Pump Inhibitors

Generic Name	Metformin Hydrochloride
Brand Name	Glucophage®, Glucophage XR®
Drug Class	Antidiabetic
Indication	Used for lowering of blood sugar in Type II diabetes, sometimes used in combination with insulin or non-insulin dependent diabetes mellitus (NIDDM)

FUROSEMIDE

. . . .

POTASSIUM CHLORIDE (ORAL)

. . . .

GABAPENTIN

PHARMACY TECHNICIAN FLASH REVIEW

Generic Name	Furosemide
Brand Name	Lasix®
Drug Class	Diuretic—loop
Indication	Treatment of edema and hypertension

· ·

Generic Name	Potassium Chloride
Brand Name	K-Dur®, Klor-Con®, Micro-K®, many others
Drug Class	Potassium supplement (oral)
Indication	Treatment and prevention of potassium deficiency (hypokalemia)

· ·

Generic Name	Gabapentin
Brand Name	Neurontin®
Drug Class	Antiepileptic
Indication	Used as an adjunct in the treatment of partial seizures; can also be used for neuralgia (nerve pain) and restless leg syndrome (RLS)

PHARMACY TECHNICIAN FLASH REVIEW

AMLODIPINE BESYLATE

. . . .

ALBUTEROL SULFATE

. . . .

ALPRAZOLAM

Generic Name	**Amlodipine Besylate**
Brand Name	Norvasc®
Drug Class	Antihypertensive—calcium channel blocker
Indication	Treatment of hypertension, can also be used for treatment of angina

Generic Name	**Albuterol Sulfate**
Brand Name	Proair HFA®, Proventil HFA®, Ventolin HFA®
Drug Class	Bronchodilator, antiasthmatic (inhalation)
Indication	Treatment of asthma and bronchospasms

Generic Name	**Alprazolam**
Brand Name	Xanax®, Xanax XR®
Drug Class	Antianxiety—benzodiazepine
Indication	Treatment of anxiety and panic disorders
Controlled Substance	C-IV

CITALOPRAM HYDROBROMIDE

· ·

RANITIDINE HYDROCHLORIDE

· ·

ZOLPIDEM TARTRATE

Generic Name	Citalopram Hydrobromide
Brand Name	Celexa®
Drug Class	Antidepressant—Selective Serotonin Reuptake Inhibitor (SSRI)
Indication	Treatment of depression

. . . .

Generic Name	Ranitidine Hydrochloride
Brand Name	Zantac®
Drug Class	Antiulcer agent—H_2 receptor blocker
Indication	Treatment of Gastroesophageal Reflux Disease (GERD), ulcers, and other hypersecretory conditions.
Hint	-tidine ending for H_2 receptor blockers

. . . .

Generic Name	Zolpidem Tartrate
Brand Name	Ambien®, Ambien CR®
Drug Class	Sedative, hypnotic
Indication	Treatment of insomnia
Controlled Substance	C-IV

ATORVASTATIN CALCIUM

. . . .

HYDROCHLOROTHIAZIDE (HCTZ)

. . . .

TRAMADOL HYDROCHLORIDE

Generic Name	Atorvastatin Calcium
Brand Name	Lipitor®
Drug Class	Antihyperlipidemic—HMG-CoA Reductase Inhibitor (statin)
Indication	Treatment of high cholesterol
Hint	-statin ending for HMG-CoA Reductase Inhibitors

. . . .

Generic Name	Hydrochlorothiazide (HCTZ)
Brand Name	HydroDiuril®, Esidrix®
Drug Class	Diuretic—thiazide
Indication	Treatment of edema and hypertension

. . . .

Generic Name	Tramadol Hydrochloride
Brand Name	Ultram®, Ryzolt®, Ultram ER®
Drug Class	Analgesic
Indication	Management of moderate to moderately severe pain

METOPROLOL TARTATE

. . . .

TRAZODONE HYDROCHLORIDE

. . . .

DULOXETINE HYDROCHLORIDE

Generic Name	Metoprolol Tartate
Brand Name	Lopressor®
Drug Class	Antihypertensive—beta blocker
Indication	Treatment of hypertension (high blood pressure) and angina
Hint	–lol ending for beta blockers

. . . .

Generic Name	Trazodone Hydrochloride
Brand Name	Desyrel®
Drug Class	Antidepressant
Indication	Treatment of depression

. . . .

Generic Name	Duloxetine Hydrochloride
Brand Name	Cymbalta®
Drug Class	Antidepressant—Selective Serotonin and Norepinephrine Reuptake Inhibitor (SNRI)
Indication	Treatment of depression; also used for treatment of fibromyalgia, diabetic neuropathy, and other chronic pain

CARVEDILOL

· ·

WARFARIN SODIUM

· ·

CLOPIDOGREL BISULFATE

Generic Name	Carvedilol
Brand Name	Coreg®, Coreg CR®
Drug Class	Antihypertensive—beta blocker
Indication	Treatment of hypertension (high blood pressure)
Hint	–lol ending for beta blockers

. . . .

Generic Name	Warfarin Sodium
Brand Name	Coumadin®, Jantoven®
Drug Class	Anticoagulant
Indication	Prevention of blood clots

. . . .

Generic Name	Clopidogrel Bisulfate
Brand Name	Plavix®
Drug Class	Platelet inhibitor
Indication	Prevention of blood clots

CLONAZEPAM

. . . .

MONTELUKAST SODIUM

. . . .

CYCLOBENZAPRINE HYDROCHLORIDE

PHARMACY TECHNICIAN FLASH REVIEW

Generic Name	Clonazepam
Brand Name	Klonopin®
Drug Class	Antiepileptic (benzodiazepine)
Indication	Treatment of seizures
Controlled Substance	C-IV
Hint	Most benzodiazepines end in –am.

Generic Name	Montelukast Sodium
Brand Name	Singulair®
Drug Class	Antiasthmatic—Leukotriene Inhibitor
Indication	Treatment of asthma, bronchospasms, and seasonal allergies

Generic Name	Cyclobenzaprine Hydrochloride
Brand Name	Flexeril®, Amrix®, Fexmid®
Drug Class	Muscle relaxant
Indication	Treatment of muscle spasms

SERTRALINE HYDROCHLORIDE

. . . .

INSULIN GLARGINE

. . . .

METOPROLOL SUCCINATE

Generic Name	Sertraline Hydrochloride
Brand Name	Zoloft®
Drug Class	Antidepressant—Selective Serotonin Reuptake Inhibitor (SSRI)
Indication	Treatment of depression

· ·

Generic Name	Insulin Glargine
Brand Name	Lantus®
Drug Class	Antidiabetic
Indication	Treatment of insulin-dependent (type I) diabetes or type II diabetes not properly controlled

· ·

Generic Name	Metoprolol Succinate
Brand Name	Toprol XL®
Drug Class	Antihypertensive—beta blocker
Indication	Treatment of hypertension (high blood pressure) and angina
Hint	–lol ending for beta blockers

QUETIAPINE FUMERATE

. . . .

LOVASTATIN

. . . .

ESOMEPRAZOLE MAGNESIUM

Generic Name	Quetiapine Fumerate
Brand Name	Seroquel®
Drug Class	Antipsychotic—atypical
Indication	Treatment of schizophrenia and bipolar disorder

. . . .

Generic Name	Lovastatin
Brand Name	Mevacor®
Drug Class	Antihyperlipidemic—HMG-CoA Reductase Inhibitor (statin)
Indication	Treatment of high cholesterol
Hint	-statin ending for HMG-CoA Reductase Inhibitors for high cholesterol

. . . .

Generic Name	Esomeprazole Magnesium
Brand Name	Nexium®
Drug Class	Antiulcer agent—Proton Pump Inhibitor (PPI)
Indication	Treatment of Gastroesophageal Reflux Disease (GERD), ulcers, and other hypersecretory conditions
Hint	-prazole ending for generic Proton Pump Inhibitors

FLUTICASONE PROPIONATE WITH SALMETEROL XINAFOATE

. . . .

FLUOXETINE HYDROCHLORIDE

. . . .

PROMETHAZINE HYDROCHLORIDE WITH CODEINE PHOSPHATE

Generic Name	Fluticasone Propionate with Salmeterol Xinafoate
Brand Name	Advair®
Drug Class	Antiasthmatic (inhalation)
Indication	Treatment of asthma and COPD

Generic Name	Fluoxetine Hydrochloride
Brand Name	Prozac®, Sarafem®
Drug Class	Antidepressant—Selective Serotonin Reuptake Inhibitor (SSRI)
Indication	Treatment of depression disorders (Sarafem® used to treat PMDD)

Generic Name	Promethazine Hydrochloride with Codeine Phosphate
Brand Name	Phenergan® with codeine
Drug Class	Antitussive
Indication	Treatment of cough
Controlled Substance	C-V

PHARMACY TECHNICIAN FLASH REVIEW

FLUTICASONE PROPIONATE

· ·

BUPROPION HYDROCHLORIDE

· ·

AMITRIPTYLINE HYDROCHLORIDE

Generic Name	Fluticasone Propionate
Brand Name	Flonase®, Veramyst®
Drug Class	Antiallergy-steroid (nasal spray)
Indication	Treatment of seasonal allergies and rhinitis

Generic Name	Bupropion Hydrochloride
Brand Name	Wellbutrin®, Wellbutrin SR®, and Wellbutrin XL®, Zyban®
Drug Class	Antidepressant
Indication	Treatment of depression; Zyban® is for smoking cessation

Generic Name	Amitriptyline Hydrochloride
Brand Name	Elavil® (brand name not available in the United States)
Drug Class	Tricyclic antidepressant (TCA)
Indication	Treatment of depression

LORAZEPAM

. . . .

MELOXICAM

. . . .

OXYCODONE HYDROCHLORIDE WITH ACETAMINOPHEN

PHARMACY TECHNICIAN FLASH REVIEW

Generic Name	Lorazepam
Brand Name	Ativan®
Drug Class	Antianxiety—benzodiazepine
Indication	Treatment of anxiety
Hint	Most benzodiazepines end in -am.

Generic Name	Meloxicam
Brand Name	Mobic®
Drug Class	NSAID (Nonsteroidal anti-inflammatory drug)
Indication	Relief of symptoms associated with arthritis

Generic Name	Oxycodone Hydrochloride with Acetaminophen
Brand Name	Percocet®, Roxicet®, Endocet®, Tylox®, Xolox®, Primalev®
Drug Class	Opioid analgesic
Indication	Relief of moderate to moderately severe pain
Controlled Substance	C-II

PHARMACY TECHNICIAN FLASH REVIEW

DILTIAZEM HYDROCHLORIDE

. . . .

ATENOLOL

. . . .

ESCITALOPRAM OXALATE

Generic Name	Diltiazem Hydrochloride
Brand Name	Cardizem®, Cardizem SR®, Cardizem CD®, Cardizem LA®, Cartia XT®, Dilacor XR®, Dilt-CD®, Dilt-XR®, Diltia XT®, Diltzac®, Taztia XT®, Tiazac®
Drug Class	Antihypertensive—calcium channel blocker
Indication	Treatment of hypertension; can also be used for treatment of angina

Generic Name	Atenolol
Brand Name	Tenormin®
Drug Class	Antihypertensive—beta blocker
Indication	Treatment of hypertension (high blood pressure)
Hint	–lol ending for beta blockers

Generic Name	Escitalopram Oxalate
Brand Name	Lexapro®
Drug Class	Antidepressant—Selective Serotonin Reuptake Inhibitor (SSRI)
Indication	Treatment of depression

OXYCODONE HYDROCHLORIDE

. . . .

TOPIRAMATE

. . . .

IPRATROPIUM BROMIDE WITH ALBUTEROL SULFATE

Generic Name	Oxycodone Hydrochloride
Brand Name	Oxycontin®, Roxicodone®
Drug Class	Opioid analgesic
Indication	Relief of moderate to moderately severe pain
Controlled Substance	C-II

· ·

Generic Name	Topiramate
Brand Name	Topamax®
Drug Class	Antiepileptic, anticonvulsant
Indication	Treatment of seizures, also used for prophylaxis of migraines

· ·

Generic Name	Ipratropium Bromide with Albuterol Sulfate
Brand Name	Combivent® (MDI Inhaler) and Duoneb® (solution for inhalation)
Drug Class	Antiasthmatic—combination bronchodialator
Indication	Treatment of COPD
Special Considerations	Contraindicated in patients with peanut allergies

TIOTROPIUM BROMIDE

. . . .

PREDNISONE

. . . .

VENLAFAXINE HYDROCHLORIDE

PHARMACY TECHNICIAN FLASH REVIEW

Generic Name	**Tiotropium Bromide**
Brand Name	Spiriva®
Drug Class	Antiasthmatic (inhalation)
Indication	Treatment of COPD, including chronic bronchitis and emphysema

Generic Name	**Prednisone**
Brand Name	Deltasone®
Drug Class	Anti-inflammatory (corticosteroid)
Indication	Treatment of inflammatory conditions

Generic Name	**Venlafaxine Hydrochloride**
Brand Name	Effexor®
Drug Class	Antidepressant—SNRI
Indication	Treatment of depression

CLONIDINE HYDROCHLORIDE

· ·

ARIPIPRAZOLE

· ·

LISINOPRIL WITH HYDROCHLOROTHIAZIDE

PHARMACY TECHNICIAN FLASH REVIEW

Generic Name	Clonidine Hydrochloride
Brand Name	Catapres®
Drug Class	Antihypertensive
Indication	Treatment of hypertension

Generic Name	Aripiprazole
Brand Name	Abilify®
Drug Class	Antipsychotic—atypical
Indication	Treatment of schizophrenia and bipolar disorder

Generic Name	Lisinipril with Hydrochlorothiazide
Brand Name	Prinizide®, Zestoretic®
Drug Class	Antihypertensive—combination ACE inhibitor and diuretic
Indication	Treatment of hypertension

MORPHINE SULFATE

. . . .

FENOFIBRATE

. . . .

ROSUVASTATIN CALCIUM

Generic Name	**Morphine Sulfate**
Brand Name	MS Contin®, Kadian®, Avinza®, Oramorph SR®, MSIR®
Drug Class	Opioid analgesic
Indication	Management of moderate to severe pain
Controlled Substance	C-II

· ·

Generic Name	Fenofibrate
Brand Name	Tricor®
Drug Class	Antihyperlipidemic
Indication	Treatment of high cholesterol

· ·

Generic Name	**Rosuvastatin Calcium**
Brand Name	Crestor®
Drug Class	Antihyperlipidemic—HMG-CoA Reductase Inhibitor (statin)
Indication	Treatment of high cholesterol
Hint	*-statin* ending for HMG-CoA Reductase Inhibitors

PHARMACY TECHNICIAN FLASH REVIEW

AZITHROMYCIN DIHYDRATE

. . . .

PRAVASTATIN SODIUM

. . . .

NAPROXEN

Generic Name	**Azithromycin Dihydrate**
Brand Name	Zithromax®, Z-Pak®, Z-max®
Drug Class	Antibiotic—macrolide
Indication	Treatment of lower and upper respiratory tract infections, bacterial sinusitis, acute otitis media, and other bacterial infections
Hint	-*mycin* ending for macrolide antibiotics

Generic Name	**Pravastatin Calcium**
Brand Name	Pravachol®
Drug Class	Antihyperlipidemic—HMG-CoA Reductase Inhibitor (statin)
Indication	Treatment of high cholesterol
Hint	-*statin* ending for HMG-CoA Reductase Inhibitors

Generic Name	**Naproxen**
Brand Name	Naprosyn®, EC-Naprosyn®, Aleve®
Drug Class	Nonsteroidal anti-inflammatory drug (NSAID)
Indication	Treatment of mild to moderate pain, including pain from arthritis and other inflammatory conditions

TAMSULOSIN HYDROCHLORIDE

. . . .

DIVALPROEX SODIUM

. . . .

DONEPEZIL HYDROCHLORIDE

PHARMACY TECHNICIAN FLASH REVIEW

Generic Name	Tamsulosin Hydrochloride
Brand Name	Flomax®
Drug Class	Alpha blocker for Benign Prostatic Hyperplasia (BPH) treatment
Indication	Treatment of enlarged prostate

Generic Name	Divalproex Sodium
Brand Name	Depakote®, Depakote ER®, Depakote Sprinkles®
Drug Class	Antiepileptic
Indication	Treatment of seizures, bipolar disorders, and migraine prophylaxis

Generic Name	Donepezil Hydrochloride
Brand Name	Aricept®
Drug Class	Antipsychotic
Indication	Treatment of Alzheimer's dementia

IBUPROFEN

. . . .

PREGABALIN

. . . .

LAMOTRIGINE

Generic Name	Ibuprofen
Brand Name	Advil®, Motrin®
Drug Class	Nonsteroidal anti-inflammatory drug (NSAID)
Indication	Treatment of mild pain and inflammatory conditions

Generic Name	Pregabalin
Brand Name	Lyrica®
Drug Class	Anticonvulsant
Indication	Used as an adjunct in treatment of epilepsy and seizures; can also be used for neuropathic pain and fibromyalgia
Controlled Substance	C-V

Generic Name	Lamotrigine
Brand Name	Lamictal®
Drug Class	Antiepileptic-anticonvulsant
Indication	Used as an adjunct in treatment of epilepsy and seizures

ALENDRONATE SODIUM

. . . .

ISOSORBIDE MONONITRATE

. . . .

SPIRONOLACTONE

Generic Name	Alendronate Sodium
Brand Name	Fosamax®
Drug Class	Osteoporosis Agent—bisphosphonate
Indication	Treatment of osteoporosis
Hint	-dronate ending for bisphosphonates for osteoporosis

Generic Name	Isosorbide Mononitrate
Brand Name	Imdur®
Drug Class	Antianginal Agent
Indication	Treatment and prophylaxis of angina

Generic Name	Spironolactone
Brand Name	Aldactone®
Drug Class	Diuretic—potassium sparing
Indication	Treatment of edema and hypertension
Special Considerations	Should be avoided in patients on an ACE inhibitor

PHARMACY TECHNICIAN FLASH REVIEW

LOSARTAN POTASSIUM

. . . .

GLIPIZIDE

. . . .

RISPERIDONE

Generic Name	Losartan potassium
Brand Name	Cozaar®
Drug Class	Antihypertensive—Angiotensin II receptor blocker (ARB)
Indication	Treatment of hypertension
Hint	-sartan ending for all ARBs

Generic Name	Glipizide
Brand Name	Glucotrol®
Drug Class	Antidiabetic—Oral Hypoglycemic Agent
Indication	Used as an adjunct in treatment of type II diabetes

Generic Name	Risperidone
Brand Name	Risperdal®
Drug Class	Antipsychotic—atypical
Indication	Treatment of schizophrenia; can also be used for bipolar treatment and irritability associated with autism

PHARMACY TECHNICIAN FLASH REVIEW

CARISOPRODOL

. . . .

ROPINIROLE HYDROCHLORIDE

. . . .

DIAZEPAM

PHARMACY TECHNICIAN FLASH REVIEW

Generic Name	Carisoprodol
Brand Name	Soma®
Drug Class	Muscle Relaxant
Indication	Relief of musculoskeletal conditions
Controlled Substance	C-IV

. . . .

Generic Name	Ropinirole Hydrochloride
Brand Name	Requip®, Requip XL®
Drug Class	Antiparkinson Agent
Indication	Treatment of signs and symptoms of Parkinson's disease as well as restless leg syndrome (RLS)

. . . .

Generic Name	Diazepam
Brand Name	Valium®
Drug Class	Antianxiety—Benzodiazepine
Indication	Management of anxiety disorders
Controlled Substance	C-IV
Hint	Many benzodiazepine generic names end in -am

Generic Name	Carisoprodol
Brand Name	Soma®
Drug Class	Muscle Relaxant
Indication	Relief of musculoskeletal conditions
Controlled Substance	C-IV

. . . .

Generic Name	Ropinirole Hydrochloride
Brand Name	Requip®, Requip XL®
Drug Class	Antiparkinson Agent
Indication	Treatment of signs and symptoms of Parkinson's disease as well as restless leg syndrome (RLS)

. . . .

Generic Name	Diazepam
Brand Name	Valium®
Drug Class	Antianxiety—Benzodiazepine
Indication	Management of anxiety disorders
Controlled Substance	C-IV
Hint	Many benzodiazepine generic names end in -am

CARISOPRODOL

· ·

ROPINIROLE HYDROCHLORIDE

· ·

DIAZEPAM

PIOGLITAZONE HYDROCHLORIDE

. . . .

MEMANTINE HYDROCHLORIDE

. . . .

METOCLOPRAMIDE HYDROCHLORIDE

PHARMACY TECHNICIAN FLASH REVIEW

Generic Name	Pioglitazone Hydrochloride
Brand Name	Actos®
Drug Class	Antidiabetic—Oral Hypoglycemic Agent
Indication	Used as an adjunct in treatment of type II diabetes

Generic Name	Memantine Hydrochloride
Brand Name	Namenda®
Drug Class	Agent for Alzheimer's Dementia
Indication	Treatment for Alzheimer's dementia

Generic Name	Metoclopramide Hydrochloride
Brand Name	Reglan®
Drug Class	Antiemetic
Indication	Prevention of nausea and vomiting

BACLOFEN

. . . .

FOLIC ACID

. . . .

AMOXICILLIN TRIHYDRATE

Generic Name	Baclofen
Brand Name	Lioresal®
Drug Class	Muscle Relaxant
Indication	Used to control muscle spasms, especially those associated with multiple sclerosis

. . . .

Generic Name	Folic Acid
Brand Name	Folate®
Drug Class	Vitamin
Indication	Treatment of anemia or folic acid deficiency

. . . .

Generic Name	Amoxicillin Trihydrate
Brand Name	Amoxil®, Trimox®
Drug Class	Antibiotic—Penicillin
Indication	Treatment of bacterial infections of the ear, nose, throat, skin, and respiratory tract, and for the treatment of gonorrhea
Hint	-cillin ending for penicillins

PHARMACY TECHNICIAN FLASH REVIEW

AMPHETAMINE AND DEXTROAMPHETAMINE SALTS

. . . .

BUSPIRONE HYDROCHLORIDE

. . . .

GLYBURIDE

Generic Name	Amphetamine and Dextroamphetamine Salts
Brand Name	Adderall®
Drug Class	CNS Stimulant
Indication	Treatment of attention deficit disorder with hyperactivity (ADHD) and narcolepsy
Controlled Substance	C-II

Generic Name	Buspirone Hydrochloride
Brand Name	Buspar®
Drug Class	Antianxiety Agent
Indication	Treatment of anxiety

Generic Name	Glyburide
Brand Name	Diabeta®, Micronase®
Drug Class	Antidiabetic—Oral Hypoglycemic
Indication	Used as an adjunct in the treatment of type II diabetes

PROMETHAZINE HCl

. . . .

LEVETIRACETAM

. . . .

SULFAMETHOXAZOLE WITH TRIMETHOPRIM

Generic Name	Promethazine HCl
Brand Name	Phenergan®
Drug Class	Antihistamine
Indication	Treatment of seasonal allergies, nausea and vomiting, and preoperative sedation

Generic Name	Levetiracetam
Brand Name	Keppra®
Drug Class	Antiepileptic, Anticonvulsant
Indication	Used as an adjunct in the treatment of partial seizures

Generic Name	Sulfamethoxazole with Trimethoprim
Brand Name	Bactrim®, Septra®, SMZ-TMP DS®
Drug Class	Antibacterial—sulfonamide
Indication	Used for the treatment of urinary tract infections and other bacterial infections
Hint	*Sulfa-* beginning for all sulfa antibacterials

PANTOPRAZOLE SODIUM

. . . .

DIGOXIN

. . . .

LIDOCAINE

Generic Name	Pantoprazole Sodium
Brand Name	Protonix®
Drug Class	Antiulcer Agent—Proton Pump Inhibitor (PPI)
Indication	Treatment of Gastroesophageal Reflux Disease (GERD), ulcers, and other hypersecretory conditions
Hint	-prazole ending for Proton Pump Inhibitors

Generic Name	Digoxin
Brand Name	Digitek®, Lanoxin®, Lanoxicaps®
Drug Class	Cardiac Glycoside (Inotropic Agent)
Indication	Used for treatment of heart failure, atrial fibrillation and flutter, and tachycardia

Generic Name	Lidocaine
Brand Name	Lidoderm®
Drug Class	Topical Analgesic (transdermal)
Indication	Relief of pain associated with neuralgia

TOLTERODINE TARTRATE

. . . .

TRIAMTERENE WITH HYDROCHLOROTHIAZIDE

. . . .

PAROXETINE HYDROCHLORIDE

Generic Name	Tolterodine Tartrate
Brand Name	Detrol®, Detrol LA®
Drug Class	Urinary Antispasmodic
Indication	Treatment of overactive bladder and urinary urgency and urge incontinence

Generic Name	Triamterene with Hydrochlorothiazide
Brand Name	Diazide® (capsules), Maxzide® (tablets)
Drug Class	Diuretic: Combination—potassium sparing and thiazide
Indication	Treatment of edema and hypertension

Generic Name	Paroxetine Hydrochloride
Brand Name	Paxil®, Paxil CR®, Pexeva®
Drug Class	Antidepressant
Indication	Treatment of depression, can also be used for obsessive compulsive disorder, panic disorder, and social anxiety disorder

PHARMACY TECHNICIAN FLASH REVIEW

HYDROXYZINE HYDROCHLORIDE

. . . .

DICYCLOMINE HYDROCHLORIDE

. . . .

GLIMEPIRIDE

Generic Name	Hydroxyzine Hydrochloride
Brand Name	Atarax®
Drug Class	Antihistamine
Indication	Treatment of pruritus and other allergic conditions; can also be used to treat anxiety through sedating effects

Generic Name	Dicyclomine Hydrochloride
Brand Name	Bentyl®
Drug Class	GI Antispasmodic
Indication	Treatment of irritable bowel syndrome

Generic Name	Glimepiride
Brand Name	Amaryl®
Drug Class	Antidiabetic—oral hypoglycemic
Indication	Used as an adjunct in the treatment of type II diabetes

CELECOXIB

. . . .

INSULIN ASPART (rDNA ORIGIN)

. . . .

ESTROGENS (CONJUGATED)

Generic Name	Celecoxib
Brand Name	Celebrex®
Drug Class	Nonsteroidal Anti-Inflammatory Drug (NSAID)—COX-2 inhibitor
Indication	Treatment of symptoms of osteoarthritis, rheumatoid arthritis, and other inflammatory conditions

Generic Name	Insulin Aspart (rDNA origin)
Brand Name	Novolog®
Drug Class	Antidiabetic
Indication	Treatment of insulin-dependent (type I) diabetes or type II diabetes not properly controlled, may be used in conjunction with long-acting insulin

Generic Name	Estrogens (Conjugated)
Brand Name	Premarin®, Cenestin®, Enjuvia®
Drug Class	Estrogen Hormone
Indication	Treatment of symptoms of menopause, female hypogonadism, and prostate cancer

HYDROXYZINE PAMOATE

. . . .

TIZANIDINE HYDROCHLORIDE

. . . .

METHYLPHENIDATE HYDROCHLORIDE

Generic Name	Hydroxyzine Pamoate
Brand Name	Vistaril®
Drug Class	Antihistamine
Indication	Treatment of anxiety, chronic uticaria, and atopic dermatitis; also used as a sedative

· ·

Generic Name	Tizanidine Hydrochloride
Brand Name	Zanaflex®
Drug Class	Muscle Relaxant
Indication	Management of muscle spasticity

· ·

Generic Name	Methylphenidate Hydrochloride
Brand Name	Ritalin®, Metadate ER®, Concerta®
Drug Class	CNS Stimulant
Indication	Treatment of ADHD and narcolepsy
Controlled Substance	C-II

CIPROFLOXACIN HYDROCHLORIDE

. . . .

LANSOPRAZOLE

. . . .

EZETIMIBE

Generic Name	Ciprofloxacin Hydrochloride
Brand Name	Cipro®, Cipro XR®
Drug Class	Antibiotic—fluoroquinolone
Indication	Treatment of bacterial infections such as those that cause UTI, infectious diarrhea, and gonorrhea
Hint	-floxacin ending for fluoroquinolones

Generic Name	Lansoprazole
Brand Name	Prevacid®
Drug Class	Antiulcer Agent—Proton Pump Inhibitor (PPI)
Indication	Treatment of Gastroesophageal Reflux Disease (GERD), ulcers, and other hypersecretory conditions
Hint	-prazole ending for Proton Pump Inhibitors

Generic Name	Ezetimibe
Brand Name	Zetia®
Drug Class	Antihyperlipidemic
Indication	Treatment of high cholesterol

PHARMACY TECHNICIAN FLASH REVIEW

PROPRANOLOL HYDROCHLORIDE

· ·

BUDESONIDE AND FORMOTEROL FUMARATE DIHYDRATE

· ·

FENTANYL

Generic Name	Propranolol Hydrochloride
Brand Name	Inderal®, Inderal LA®, InnoPran XL®
Drug Class	Antihypertensive—beta blocker
Indication	Treatment of hypertension (high blood pressure)
Hint	–lol ending for beta blockers

Generic Name	Budesonide and Formoterol Fumarate Dihydrate
Brand Name	Symbicort®
Drug Class	Antiasthmatic (inhalation)
Indication	Treatment of asthma and COPD

Generic Name	Fentanyl
Brand Name	Duragesic®
Drug Class	Opioid Analgesic (transdermal)
Indication	Management of chronic pain
Controlled Substance	C-II

PHARMACY TECHNICIAN FLASH REVIEW

NYSTATIN

· ·

DOXYCYCLINE HYCLATE

· ·

INSULIN LISPRO

Generic Name	Nystatin
Brand Name	Nystop® (powder), Mycostatin® (cream, suspension)
Drug Class	Antifungal
Indication	Treatment of fungal infections including oral candidiasis (thrush)

Generic Name	Doxycycline Hyclate
Brand Name	Vibramycin®
Drug Class	Antibiotic—tetracycline
Indication	Treatment of bacterial infections, including syphilis, gonorrhea, acne, and prophylaxis of malaria
Hint	-cycline ending for tetracyclines

Generic Name	Insulin Lispro
Brand Name	Humalog®
Drug Class	Antidiabetic
Indication	Treatment of insulin-dependent (type I) diabetes or type II diabetes not properly controlled

CARBIDOPA WITH LEVODOPA

. . . .

VALSARTAN

. . . .

FAMOTIDINE

PHARMACY TECHNICIAN FLASH REVIEW

Generic Name	Carbidopa with Levodopa
Brand Name	Sinemet®
Drug Class	Antiparkinson Agent
Indication	Treatment of symptoms of Parkinson's disease

Generic Name	Valsartan
Brand Name	Diovan®
Drug Class	Antihypertensive—Angiotensin II receptor blocker (ARB)
Indication	Treatment of hypertension
Hint	-sartan generic ending for ARBs

Generic Name	Famotidine
Brand Name	Pepcid®
Drug Class	Antiulcer agent—H$_2$ receptor blocker
Indication	Treatment of Gastroesophageal Reflux Disease (GERD) and ulcers
Hint	-tidine generic ending for H$_2$ receptor blockers

SITAGLIPTIN PHOSPHATE

. . . .

ESZOPICLONE

. . . .

TEMAZEPAM

Generic Name	Sitagliptin Phosphate
Brand Name	Januvia®
Drug Class	Antidiabetic
Indication	Treatment of type 2 diabetes

Generic Name	Eszopiclone
Brand Name	Lunesta®
Drug Class	Sedative
Indication	Treatment of insomnia
Controlled Substance	C-IV

Generic Name	Temazepam
Brand Name	Restoril®
Drug Class	Sedative
Indication	Treatment of insomnia
Controlled Substance	C-IV

VERAPAMIL HYDROCHLORIDE

. . . .

CHLORPHENIRAMINE WITH HYDROCODONE

. . . .

ENALAPRIL MALEATE

Generic Name	Verapamil Hydrochloride
Brand Name	Calan®, Isoptin®, Verelen®
Drug Class	Antihypertensive—calcium channel blocker
Indication	Treatment of hypertension and angina

Generic Name	Chlorpheniramine with Hydrocodone
Brand Name	Tussionex®
Drug Class	Antitussive
Indication	Treatment of cough
Controlled Substance	C-III

Generic Name	Enalapril Maleate
Brand Name	Vasotec®
Drug Class	Antihypertensive—ACE inhibitor
Indication	Treatment of high blood pressure
Hint	ACE inhibitor generic names end in -pril

SOLIFENACIN SUCCINATE

. . . .

ESTRADIOL

. . . .

PRAMIPEXOLE DIHYDROCHLORIDE

Generic Name	Solifenacin Succinate
Brand Name	Vesicare®
Drug Class	Urinary Antispasmodic
Indication	Treatment of overactive bladder and urinary incontinence

Generic Name	Estradiol
Brand Name	Vivelle-Dot®
Drug Class	Hormone Replacement (topical)
Indication	Treatment of symptoms associated with menopause or estrogen replacement due to ovarian failure

Generic Name	Pramipexole Dihydrochloride
Brand Name	Mirapex®
Drug Class	Antiparkinson Agent
Indication	Treatment of symptoms of Parkinson's disease

CARBAMAZEPINE

. . . .

PHENYTOIN SODIUM (EXTENDED)

. . . .

LEVALBUTEROL HYDROCHLORIDE

PHARMACY TECHNICIAN FLASH REVIEW

Generic Name	Carbamazepine
Brand Name	Tegretol®, Carbatrol®, Epitol®, Equetro®, Tegretol XR®
Drug Class	Anticonvulsant
Indication	Treatment of seizures and nerve pain, may also be used for treatment of bipolar disorder

Generic Name	Phenytoin Sodium (Extended)
Brand Name	Dilantin®, Phenytek®
Drug Class	Antiepileptic—Anticonvulsant
Indication	Control of seizures

Generic Name	Levalbuterol Hydrochloride
Brand Name	Xopenex®
Drug Class	Brochodialator—Antiasthmatic
Indication	Treatment of asthma and COPD

CEPHALEXIN MONOHYDRATE

. . . .

DESVENLAFAXINE

. . . .

MOMETASONE FUROATE MONOHYDRATE

PHARMACY TECHNICIAN FLASH REVIEW

Generic Name	**Cephalexin Monohydrate**
Brand Name	Keflex®
Drug Class	Antibiotic—cephalosporin
Indication	Treatment of bacterial infections, such as those that cause otitis media, strep throat, UTIs, and skin infections

• •

Generic Name	**Desvenlafaxine**
Brand Name	Pristiq®
Drug Class	Antidepressant—serotonin and norepinephrine reuptake inhibitor (SNRI)
Indication	Treatment of depression

• •

Generic Name	**Mometasone Furoate Monohydrate**
Brand Name	Nasonex®
Drug Class	Antiallergy agent (nasal spray)—steroid
Indication	Treatment and prophylaxis of nasal allergy symptoms

ZIPRASIDONE HYDROCHLORIDE

. . . .

NIACIN (EXTENDED RELEASE)

. . . .

FLUCONAZOLE

Generic Name	Ziprasidone Hydrochloride
Brand Name	Geodon®
Drug Class	Antipsychotic
Indication	Treatment of schizophrenia

Generic Name	Niacin (Extended Release)
Brand Name	Niacin®, Niacin SR®, Niacor®, Niaspan ER®, Slo-Niacin®
Drug Class	Antihyperlipidemic
Indication	Treatment of high cholesterol, may also be used to treat coronary artery disease (atherosclerosis)

Generic Name	Fluconazole
Brand Name	Diflucan®
Drug Class	Antifungal
Indication	Treatment of vaginal candidiasis and other fungal infections

PHARMACY TECHNICIAN FLASH REVIEW

GEMFIBROZIL

. . . .

LITHIUM CARBONATE

. . . .

TRIAMCINOLONE ACETONIDE

Generic Name	Gemfibrozil
Brand Name	Lopid®
Drug Class	Antihyperlipidemic
Indication	Treatment of high cholesterol

Generic Name	Lithium Carbonate
Brand Name	Eskalith®, Lithobid®, Lithonate®
Drug Class	Antipsychotic
Indication	Treatment of bipolar disorder

Generic Name	Triamcinolone Acetonide
Brand Name	Kenalog®, Cinolar®, Trianex®, Triderm®
Drug Class	Corticosteroid (topical)
Indication	Relief of inflammatory and pruritic symptoms

PHARMACY TECHNICIAN FLASH REVIEW

DOXAZOSIN MESYLATE

. . . .

FLUTICASONE PROPIONATE

. . . .

OLMESARTAN MEDOXOMIL

Generic Name	Doxazosin Mesylate
Brand Name	Cardura®, Cardura XL®
Drug Class	Antihypertensive/Prostate—anti-inflammatory
Indication	Treatment of high blood pressure and benign prostatic hyperplasia (BPH)

Generic Name	Fluticasone Propionate
Brand Name	Flovent®, Flovent Diskus®, Flovent HFA®
Drug Class	Antiasthmatic—steroid
Indication	Treatment for the prevention of asthma attacks

Generic Name	Olmesartan Medoxomil
Brand Name	Benicar®
Drug Class	Antihypertensive—Angiotensin II receptor blocker (ARB)
Indication	Treatment of hypertension
Hint	-sartan generic ending for ARBs

BUTALBITAL, ACETAMINOPHEN, AND CAFFEINE

· ·

AMOXICILLIN WITH CLAVULANATE POTASSIUM

· ·

ACETAMINOPHEN WITH CODEINE PHOSPHATE

PHARMACY TECHNICIAN FLASH REVIEW

Generic Name	Butalbital, Acetaminophen, and Caffeine
Brand Name	Fioricet®
Drug Class	Analgesic
Indication	Treatment of headache

Generic Name	Amoxicillin with Clavulanate Potassium
Brand Name	Augmentin®, Augmentin ES-600®, Augmentin XR®
Drug Class	Antibiotic—penicillin
Indication	Treatment of bacterial infections, including sinusitis and otitis media

Generic Name	Acetaminophen with Codeine Phosphate
Brand Name	Tylenol with codeine®
Drug Class	Opioid Analgesic
Indication	Treatment of mild to moderate pain
Controlled Substance	C-III

INSULIN DETEMIR

. . . .

VALSARTAN WITH HYDROCHLOROTHIAZIDE

. . . .

OXCARBAZEPINE

Generic Name	Insulin Detemir
Brand Name	Levemir®
Drug Class	Antidiabetic
Indication	Treatment of insulin-dependent (type I) diabetes or type II diabetes not properly controlled

Generic Name	Valsartan with Hydrochlorothiazide
Brand Name	Diovan-HCT®
Drug Class	Antihypertensive (combination ARB and diuretic)
Indication	Treatment of hypertension

Generic Name	Oxcarbazepine
Brand Name	Trileptal®
Drug Class	Antiepileptic—Anticonvulsant
Indication	Treatment of seizures

ONDANSETRON HYDROCHLORIDE

. . . .

EZETIMIBE WITH SIMVASTATIN

. . . .

LOSARTAN POTASSIUM WITH HYDROCHLOROTHIAZIDE

PHARMACY TECHNICIAN FLASH REVIEW

Generic Name	Ondansetron Hydrochloride
Brand Name	Zofran®, Zofran ODT®
Drug Class	Antiemetic
Indication	Prevention of nausea and vomiting usually caused by cancer treatment

Generic Name	Ezetimibe with Simvastatin
Brand Name	Vytorin®
Drug Class	Antihyperlipidemic
Indication	Treatment of high cholesterol

Generic Name	Losartan Potassium with Hydrochlorothiazide
Brand Name	Hyzaar®
Drug Class	Antihypertensive (combination ARB and diuretic)
Indication	Treatment of hypertension

RAMIPRIL

· ·

DARIFENACIN HYDROBROMIDE

· ·

BENAZEPRIL HYDROCHLORIDE

Generic Name	Ramipril
Brand Name	Altace®
Drug Class	Antihypertensive—ACE inhibitor
Indication	Treatment of high blood pressure
Hint	ACE inhibitor generic names end in -pril

Generic Name	Darifenacin Hydrobromide
Brand Name	Enablex®
Drug Class	Urinary antispasmodic
Indication	Treatment of overactive bladder and urinary urgency and incontinence

Generic Name	Benazepril Hydrochloride
Brand Name	Lotensin®
Drug Class	Antihypertensive—ACE inhibitor
Indication	Treatment of high blood pressure
Hint	ACE inhibitor generic names end in -pril

SUMATRIPTAN SUCCINATE

. . . .

METHADONE HYDROCHLORIDE

. . . .

METAXALONE

Generic Name	Sumatriptan Succinate
Brand Name	Imitrex®
Drug Class	Antimigraneous Agent
Indication	Treatment of migraine headaches

Generic Name	Methadone Hydrochloride
Brand Name	Dolophine®
Drug Class	Opioid Analgesic
Indication	Used for relief of severe pain, and for the detoxification or temporary maintenance of narcotic addiction
Controlled Substance	C-II

Generic Name	Metaxalone
Brand Name	Skelaxin®
Drug Class	Muscle Relaxant
Indication	Treatment of painful musculoskeletal conditions

PHARMACY TECHNICIAN FLASH REVIEW

BENZONATATE

. . . .

BUMETANIDE

. . . .

DICLOFENAC SODIUM

Generic Name	Benzonatate
Brand Name	Tessalon Perles®
Drug Class	Antitussive
Indication	Relief of cough

Generic Name	Bumetanide
Brand Name	Bumex®
Drug Class	Diuretic—Loop
Indication	Treatment of edema and hypertension

Generic Name	Diclofenac Sodium
Brand Name	Voltaren®, Voltaren-XR®
Drug Class	Nonsteroidal anti-inflammatory drug (NSAID)—oral
Indication	Treatment of symptoms of osteoarthritis and rheumatoid arthritis

PHARMACY TECHNICIAN FLASH REVIEW

METHOTREXATE SODIUM

. . . .

OLANZAPINE

. . . .

NITROFURANTOIN

PHARMACY TECHNICIAN FLASH REVIEW

Generic Name	Methotrexate Sodium
Brand Name	Rheumatrex®, Trexall®
Drug Class	Antimetabolite
Indication	Treatment of specific types of cancer, management of severe rheumatoid arthritis and psoriasis

Generic Name	Olanzapine
Brand Name	Zyprexa®
Drug Class	Antipsychotic—atypical
Indication	Treatment of schizophrenia and bipolar disorder

Generic Name	Nitrofurantoin
Brand Name	Macrobid®, Macrodantin®
Drug Class	Antibacterial
Indication	Treatment of urinary tract infections (UTIs)

BENZTROPINE MESYLATE

. . . .

DIPYRIDAMOLE AND ASPIRIN

. . . .

AMLODIPINE BESYLATE WITH BENAZEPRIL HYDROCHLORIDE

Generic Name	Benztropine Mesylate
Brand Name	Cogentin®
Drug Class	Antiparkinson Agent
Indication	Treatment of the symptoms of Parkinson's disease

Generic Name	Dipyridamole and Aspirin
Brand Name	Aggrenox®
Drug Class	Antiplatelet Agent
Indication	Reduce the risk of stroke and blood clots

Generic Name	Amlodipine Besylate with Benazepril Hydrochloride
Brand Name	Lotrel®
Drug Class	Antihypertensive (combination calcium channel blocker and ACE inhibitor)
Indication	Treatment of hypertension

NIFEDIPINE

. . . .

OMEGA-3-ACID ETHYL ESTERS

. . . .

METHOCARBAMOL

Generic Name	Nifedipine
Brand Name	Procardia®, Nifedical XL®
Drug Class	Antihypertensive—calcium channel blocker
Indication	Treatment of hypertension and angina

Generic Name	Omega-3-Acid Ethyl Esters
Brand Name	Lovaza®
Drug Class	Antihyperlipidemic
Indication	Treatment of high cholesterol

Generic Name	Methocarbamol
Brand Name	Robaxin®
Drug Class	Muscle Relaxant
Indication	Relief of painful musculoskeletal conditions

ACYCLOVIR

· ·

FINASTERIDE

· ·

SUCRALFATE

Generic Name	Acyclovir
Brand Name	Zovirax®
Drug Class	Antiviral
Indication	Treatment of genital herpes, herpes zoster (shingles), and other viral infections

. . . .

Generic Name	Finasteride
Brand Name	Proscar®, Propecia®
Drug Class	Prostate—Anti-Inflammatory
Indication	Treatment of benign prostatic hyperplasia (BPH)

. . . .

Generic Name	Sucralfate
Brand Name	Carafate®
Drug Class	Antiulcer
Indication	Treatment of Gastroesophageal Reflux Disease (GERD), and prevention and treatment of ulcers

MUPIROCIN

. . . .

DICLOFENAC SODIUM

. . . .

OLOPATADINE HYDROCHLORIDE

Generic Name	Mupirocin
Brand Name	Bactroban®
Drug Class	Antibacterial (topical)
Indication	Treatment of impetigo, MRSA, and other bacterial skin infections

Generic Name	Diclofenac Sodium
Brand Name	Voltaren Gel®, Pennsaid®, Solaraze®
Drug Class	Nonsteroidal Anti-Inflammatory Drug (NSAID)—topical
Indication	Treatment of symptoms of osteoarthritis

Generic Name	Olopatadine Hydrochloride
Brand Name	Patanol®, Pataday®
Drug Class	Antiallergy (ophthalmic)
Indication	Treatment of allergic conjunctivitis

HYDROXYCHLOROQUINE SULFATE

. . . .

PROCHLORPERAZINE

. . . .

THYROID, DESSICATED

Generic Name	Hydroxychloroquine Sulfate
Brand Name	Plaquenil®
Drug Class	Antimalarial
Indication	Treatment of malaria, also used for SLE (systemic lupus erythematosus) and rheumatoid arthritis (RA)

Generic Name	Prochlorperazine
Brand Name	Compazine®
Drug Class	Antipsychotic—typical
Indication	Treatment of schizophrenia; can also be used to control severe nausea, vomiting, and excessive anxiety

Generic Name	Thyroid, dessicated
Brand Name	Armour® Thyroid
Drug Class	Thyroid hormone
Indication	Treatment of hypothyroidism

NEBIVOLOL HYDROCHLORIDE

. . . .

RALOXIFENE HYDROCHLORIDE

. . . .

VALACYCLOVIR HYDROCHLORIDE

PHARMACY TECHNICIAN FLASH REVIEW

Generic Name	Nebivolol Hydrochloride
Brand Name	Bystolic®
Drug Class	Antihypertensive—beta blocker
Indication	Treatment of hypertension (high blood pressure)
Hint	–lol generic ending for beta blockers

Generic Name	Raloxifene Hydrochloride
Brand Name	Evista®
Drug Class	Osteoporosis Agent
Indication	Treatment of osteoporosis in postmenopausal women

Generic Name	Valacyclovir Hydrochloride
Brand Name	Valtrex®
Drug Class	Antiviral
Indication	Treatment of genital herpes, herpes zoster (shingles), and cold sores (herpes labialis)

PHARMACY TECHNICIAN FLASH REVIEW

AMIODARONE

. . . .

DIPHENOXYLATE HYDROCHLORIDE WITH ATROPINE SULFATE

. . . .

NORTRIPTYLINE HYDROCHLORIDE

PHARMACY TECHNICIAN FLASH REVIEW

Generic Name	Amiodarone
Brand Name	Cordarone®, Pacerone®
Drug Class	Antiarrhythmic
Indication	Treatment of ventricular fibrillation and tachycardia

· ·

Generic Name	Diphenoxylate Hydrochloride with Atropine Sulfate
Brand Name	Lomotil®
Drug Class	Antidiarrheal
Indication	Treatment of diarrhea
Controlled Substance	C-V

· ·

Generic Name	Nortriptyline Hydrochloride
Brand Name	Pamelor®
Drug Class	Antidepressant—tricyclic
Indication	Treatment of depression

TERAZOSIN HYDROCHLORIDE

. . . .

QUINAPRIL HYDROCHLORIDE

. . . .

CLINDAMYCIN HYDROCHLORIDE

Generic Name	Terazosin Hydrochloride
Brand Name	Hytrin®
Drug Class	Antihypertensive/Prostate—Anti-inflammatory (alpha-adrenergic blocker)
Indication	Treatment of high blood pressure and benign prostatic hyperplasia (BPH)

· ·

Generic Name	Quinapril Hydrochloride
Brand Name	Accupril®
Drug Class	Antihypertensive—ACE inhibitor
Indication	Treatment of high blood pressure
Hint	ACE inhibitor generic names end in -pril

· ·

Generic Name	Clindamycin Hydrochloride
Brand Name	Cleocin®
Drug Class	Antibiotic
Indication	Treatment of serious respiratory tract infections and other serious bacterial infections; reserved for penicillin-allergic patients

METHYLPREDNISOLONE

. . . .

LEVOFLOXACIN

. . . .

THEOPHYLLINE ANHYDROUS

Generic Name	Methylprednisolone
Brand Name	Medrol®, Medrol Dosepak®
Drug Class	Anti-inflammatory (corticosteroid)
Indication	Treatment of inflammatory conditions

Generic Name	Levofloxacin
Brand Name	Levaquin®
Drug Class	Antibiotic—fluoroquinolone
Indication	Treatment of bacterial infections, such as those that cause community-acquired pneumonia, acute sinusitis, UTIs, among others
Hint	-floxacin ending for fluoroquinolones

Generic Name	Theophylline Anhydrous
Brand Name	Theo-Dur®, Theo-24®, Elixophyllin®
Drug Class	Bronchodilator
Indication	Treatment of the symptoms of asthma and chronic bronchitis

GUANFACINE HYDROCHLORIDE

. . . .

DOXEPIN HYDROCHLORIDE

. . . .

PHENTERMINE HYDROCHLORIDE

PHARMACY TECHNICIAN FLASH REVIEW

Generic Name	Guanfacine Hydrochloride
Brand Name	Intuniv®, Tenex®
Drug Class	Antihypertensive/ADHD Treatment
Indication	Treatment of hypertension and ADHD in children over 6 years old

Generic Name	Doxepin Hydrochloride
Brand Name	Sinequan®
Drug Class	Antidepressant—tricyclic
Indication	Treatment of depression

Generic Name	Phentermine Hydrochloride
Brand Name	Adipex-P®, Ionamin®
Drug Class	Weight Management
Indication	Used for weight reduction
Controlled Substance	C-III

VARENICLINE TARTRATE

· ·

AZELASTINE HYDROCHLORIDE

· ·

ZONISAMIDE

PHARMACY TECHNICIAN FLASH REVIEW

Generic Name	Varenicline Tartrate
Brand Name	Chantix®
Drug Class	Smoking Cessation Agent
Indication	To aid in the cessation of smoking

Generic Name	Azelastine Hydrochloride
Brand Name	Astelin®
Drug Class	Antiallergy Agent—antihistamine (nasal spray)
Indication	Treatment of seasonal rhinitis and allergy symptoms

Generic Name	Zonisamide
Brand Name	Zonegran®
Drug Class	Anticonvulsant
Indication	Used as an adjunct in the treatment of seizures

METOLAZONE

. . . .

TRAVOPROST

. . . .

TELMISARTAN

PHARMACY TECHNICIAN FLASH REVIEW

Generic Name	Metolazone
Brand Name	Zaroxolyn®
Drug Class	Diuretic
Indication	Treatment of edema and hypertension

Generic Name	Travoprost
Brand Name	Travatan®, Travatan Z®
Drug Class	Glaucoma Agent
Indication	Reduction of intraocular pressure in glaucoma

Generic Name	Telmisartan
Brand Name	Micardis®
Drug Class	Antihypertensive—angiotensin II receptor blocker (ARB)
Indication	Treatment of hypertension
Hint	-sartan generic ending for ARBs

**TRAMADOL HYDROCHLORIDE WITH
ACETAMINOPHEN**

. . . .

**CLOTRIMAZOLE WITH BETAMETHASONE
DIPROPIONATE**

. . . .

PHARMACY TECHNICIAN FLASH REVIEW

Generic Name	Tramadol Hydrochloride with Acetaminophen
Brand Name	Ultracet®
Drug Class	Analgesic—combination product
Indication	Management of acute pain

Generic Name	Clotrimazole with Betamethasone Dipropionate
Brand Name	Lotrisone®
Drug Class	Antifungal (topical combination product)
Indication	tinea pedis (athlete's foot), tinea cruris (jock itch), and tinea corporis (ringworm)

THIRD PARTY

. . . .

HEALTH MAINTENANCE ORGANIZATION (HMO)

. . . .

PREFERRED PROVIDER ORGANIZATION (PPO)

PHARMACY TECHNICIAN FLASH REVIEW

Another name for an insurance provider.

• •

A type of insurance plan that requires the designation of a primary care physician (PCP). Patients must first get referral from their PCP for any type of specialty services.

• •

A type of insurance plan that does not require the designation of a primary care physician (PCP), but has a network of preferred providers to select from when services are needed.

PREMIUM

· ·

DEDUCTIBLE

· ·

CO-PAYMENT

The cost of the insurance coverage paid for by the member.

· ·

The amount that must be paid each year out of pocket before benefits will kick in.

· ·

The fee a patient pays at the time of service.

COINSURANCE

. . . .

OUT OF POCKET EXPENSES

. . . .

SUBSCRIBER

A fee a patient pays for services rendered based on a percentage of the cost.

Example: If the plan pays 80% and the patient pays 20% of the cost of the services, and the prescription costs $100, then the patient's responsibility will be $20, and the insurance will pay $80.

. . . .

The total amount a patient will pay from their own money. This amount is generally regulated by the insurance company and set at a certain limit.

. . . .

Another name for the member, or person who pays for the insurance, under his or her healthcare plan.

DEPENDENT

. . . .

PERSON CODE

. . . .

MEDICARE

A person on a member's plan who is also covered by the insurance policy—an example could be a spouse or child.

. . . .

The code given to distinguish which person the service is being provided for.

Example: Member person code = 00

Spouse person code = 01

First child = 02, second = 03

. . . .

Government insurance provided to patients who are 65 or older, or younger patients with certain disabilities.

MEDICARE PART A

· ·

MEDICARE PART B

· ·

DURABLE MEDICAL EQUIPMENT (DME)

PHARMACY TECHNICIAN FLASH REVIEW

Portion of Medicare that provides coverage for inpatient hospital stays, nursing facilities, home healthcare services, and hospice care.

. . . .

Portion of Medicare that provides coverage for durable medical equipment (DME), outpatient services from hospitals, and physician services.

. . . .

Any medical equipment used to aid patients in achieving a better lifestyle.

Examples:

- cane
- walker
- wheelchair
- hospital bed
- insulin supplies
- nebulizer

MEDICARE PART C

. . . .

MEDICARE PART D

. . . .

MEDICAID

PHARMACY TECHNICIAN FLASH REVIEW

Portion of Medicare that is also known as the Medicare Advantage Plan; patients can receive benefits through a separate provider, but must be enrolled in Medicare Parts A and B to be eligible.

. . . .

Portion of Medicare that is the voluntary prescription drug coverage; patients must enroll during an eligibility period.

. . . .

Government-funded program run individually by each state for the low-income population.

TRICARE

. . . .

CHAMPVA

. . . .

WORKERS' COMPENSATION

Government health benefits program for military personnel and retirees; also includes dependents of active-duty service members.

. . . .

Health benefits program that helps pay medical expenses for the families of veterans who have been disabled because of injuries related to military experience.

. . . .

Medical coverage for an employee who is injured on the job; patient will pay no portion of prescription drug costs.

COORDINATION OF BENEFITS

. . . .

FORMULARY

. . . .

PHARMACY BENEFIT MANAGER (PBM)

PHARMACY TECHNICIAN FLASH REVIEW

When a patient has multiple insurance providers, one provider must be selected as the primary insurance and billed first. If there are unpaid claims that remain, the second insurance company can be billed, but only if there are charges remaining. This prevents duplication of reimbursement and payment.

. . . .

A list of drugs approved by the insurance company to be covered under an individual's plan.

A formulary is also a list medications approved by the P&T committee for administration to patients in a hospital or long-term care facility.

. . . .

A third-party administrator of prescription drug programs who processes and pays for all drug claims and manages the formulary for each plan.

PRIOR AUTHORIZATION

. . . .

REFILL TOO SOON

. . . .

PLAN LIMITATIONS EXCEEDED

Special approval needed before an insurance company will cover a specific medication for a patient, generally an expensive brand name drug that is not present on the formulary.

. . . .

An attempt by a member to get a prescription refilled before the insurance company permits a scheduled fill.

. . . .

An attempt by a member to fill a prescription for too large a quantity—for example, attempting to obtain a 90-day supply of a medication when only a 30-day supply is covered.

DRUG UTILIZATION REVIEW

. . . .

ADJUDICATION

. . . .

BILLER IDENTIFICATION NUMBER (BIN)

An evaluation required by OBRA to determine whether a medication is safe for the patient based on selected criteria and cost-effective measures.

· ·

Determining whether or not a drug will be covered under the insurance plan; once a prescription has been entered, it will undergo adjudication by the insurance company to determine coverage.

· ·

A unique 6-digit number identifying each third party to determine where the electronic claim should be sent.

PHARMACY AND THERAPEUTICS COMMITTEE (P & T COMMITTEE)

. . . .

PERIODIC AUTOMATIC REPLENISHMENT (PAR LEVEL)

. . . .

ROTATE STOCK

Committee comprised of nurses, physicians, pharmacists, and sometimes technicians within a hospital that meets on a regular basis to review issues related to medications, including:

- hospital formulary
  - reviewing, maintaining, and updating when necessary
- medication use evaluations (MUEs)
- discussing and investigating medication errors

· ·

The amount of stock that should be on the shelves to meet demands; when inventory falls below par levels, stock should be reordered to replenish inventory.

· ·

When new inventory arrives and is being placed onto the shelf for storage, it should be placed in order of shortest expiration date so as to use the products that expire first before those that expire last.

PARTIAL FILL

. . . .

JUST-IN-TIME PURCHASING

. . . .

WHOLESALER PURCHASING

PHARMACY TECHNICIAN FLASH REVIEW

If a pharmacy does not have a sufficient supply of a medication to fill an entire order for a patient, a partial fill may be given:

- usually a three- to five-day supply (enough to last the patient until the pharmacy receives stock from the wholesaler)

. . . .

Purchasing of inventory in quantities that just meet the demands until the next time ordering is completed.

- reduces amount of inventory
- can only be used if the pharmacy can predict the needs of patients, and if supplies are readily available
    - current drug shortages make just-in-time purchasing difficult

. . . .

Purchasing from one wholesaler as a single source of multiple manufacturers of drugs and other medical products.

- quick turnaround time for drugs when available
    - when drugs aren't available, known as **back orders**

CONTROLLED SUBSTANCE ORDERING SYSTEM (CSOS)

. . . .

REVERSE DISTRIBUTION

. . . .

STORAGE REQUIREMENTS

PHARMACY TECHNICIAN FLASH REVIEW

DEA electronic version of form 222 for ordering of controlled substances.

- pharmacies do not have to complete corresponding 222 paperwork for ordering

. . . .

Process of sending back medications when expired, damaged, or destroyed for credit from manufacturers.

. . . .

Unit	Temperature °F	Temperature °C
Freezer	−13°F to 14°F	−25°C to −10°C
Refrigerator	36°F to 46°F	2°C to 8°C
Room Temperature	59°F to 86°F	15°C to 30°C
Warmer	86°F to 104°F	30°C to 40°C

COMPUTER PHYSICIAN ORDER ENTRY (CPOE)

. . . .

ELECTRONIC MEDICATION ADMINISTRATION RECORD (EMAR)

. . . .

E-PRESCRIBING

PHARMACY TECHNICIAN FLASH REVIEW

The electronic entry of instructions from practitioners in a hospital for patient orders.

- can include orders for lab tests, pharmacy, physical therapy, and other hospital units

- gives other caregivers immediate access to patient orders and records

- helps improve workflow and compliance with documentation of patient issues

• •

Electronic documentation of administration of medications rather than a nurse or caregiver documenting on a paper chart; the patient's chart is electronic, and the system is paperless.

- helps minimize medication errors by eliminating handwriting illegibility

- helps minimize dosing problems and patient errors by utilizing bar-coding technology

• •

Direct transmission of prescriptions from physicians to the pharmacy; helps minimize errors due to illegibility in handwriting, and helps reduce the potential for forged prescriptions from drug-seeking patients.

PURE FOOD AND DRUG ACT OF 1906

· ·

FOOD, DRUG, AND COSMETIC ACT OF 1938 (FDCA)

· ·

ADULTERATED PRODUCT

Pure Food and Drug Act of 1906	
Purpose	• Prohibit interstate transportation of misbranded and adulterated food and drugs

. . . .

Food, Drug, and Cosmetic Act of 1938 (FDCA)	
Purpose	• Defined adulteration and misbranding • Created the FDA • Required manufacturers to submit new drug application (NDA) to FDA

. . . .

A product that may be contaminated, packaged under unsanitary conditions, prepared in containers that are composed of unsafe substances, have unsafe additives, or differ in strength, quality, or purity from what the drug is claiming to be.

MISBRANDED PRODUCT

. . . .

NEW DRUG APPLICATION (NDA)

. . . .

DURHAM-HUMPHREY AMENDMENT OF 1951

A product that has been labeled incorrectly, or whose label may include false or misleading statements about the ingredients of the drug.

· ·

Documentation required by the FDA to be filed with each new drug prior to marketing.

· ·

Amendment to the FDCA

Durham-Humphrey Amendment of 1951	
Purpose	• Distinguished between prescription and OTC medications • Required prescription drugs to bear the legend: "Caution: Federal Law Prohibits Dispensing Without a Prescription." • Allowed verbal prescriptions to be given over the phone • Allowed refills to be called in

LEGEND DRUGS

. . . .

OTC DRUGS (OVER THE COUNTER)

. . . .

KEFAUVER-HARRIS AMENDMENT OF 1962

PHARMACY TECHNICIAN FLASH REVIEW

Drugs that require a prescription in order to be dispensed.

· ·

Drugs that are available for purchase without a prescription.

· ·

Kefauver-Harris Amendment of 1962	
Purpose	• Requires all medications to be safe and effective • Passed in response to the thalidomide birth defects • Requires drug manufacturers to file investigational new drug application (INDA)

THALIDOMIDE

. . . .

INVESTIGATIONAL NEW DRUG APPLICATION (INDA)

. . . .

POISON PREVENTION PACKAGING ACT OF 1970

PHARMACY TECHNICIAN FLASH REVIEW

Drug given to pregnant mothers for morning sickness in the late 1950s and early 1960s.

- Babies were born with severe birth defects, and the Kefauver-Harris Amendment of 1962 was passed in response to this tragedy.

· ·

Documentation required by the FDA to be completed before drugs are tested in clinical trials on humans.

· ·

Poison Prevention Packaging Act of 1970	
Purpose	• Prevent accidental childhood poisonings from both prescription and OTC drugs

CHILD-RESISTANT CONTAINER

. . . .

EXCEPTIONS FOR CHILD-RESISTANT CONTAINERS

. . . .

OCCUPATIONAL SAFETY AND HEALTH ACT OF 1970

A container that cannot be opened by 80% of children under age 5 but can be opened by 90% of adults.

. . . .

According to the Poison Prevention Packaging Act, there are exceptions that do not require child-resistant containers.

Exceptions:

- if a patient requests a non-childproof resistant container (and signs a waiver)

- drugs dispensed to institutionalized patients or those ordered as such by a prescriber

Examples of common medication exceptions:

- sublingual nitroglycerin

- oral contraceptives

- inhalation aerosols

. . . .

Occupational Safety and Health Act of 1970	
Purpose	• To ensure a safe workplace for employees • Affects pharmacy employees by ensuring compliance for protection from air contamination, needle sticks, and hazardous chemical exposure

MATERIAL SAFETY DATA SHEETS (MSDS)

. . . .

EYEWASH

. . . .

SPILL KIT

Provided to the pharmacy about each chemical; contains important information on the hazards of particular substances, including flammability and reactivity of chemicals. Also includes information on how to store chemicals and what to do in the event of a spill or accidental ingestion.

· ·

Used for flushing contaminants from the eye after exposure to a hazardous chemical.

· ·

Provides protection in the event of a spill, in such cases as chemotherapy (cytotoxic drugs), certain antibiotics, and some radiopharmaceuticals.

COMPREHENSIVE DRUG ABUSE PREVENTION AND CONTROL ACT OF 1970 (CSA)

. . . .

CONTROLLED SUBSTANCE

. . . .

DEA NUMBER

Comprehensive Drug Abuse Prevention and Control Act of 1970 (CSA)	
Purpose	• To combat drug abuse and regulate prescription drug use of narcotics and controlled substances

. . . .

Drugs that have a high risk for physical and psychological dependence and abuse, placed into one of five schedules based on potential for abuse.

. . . .

Issued to practitioners authorized to prescribe controlled substances.

Step	Verifying a DEA number is valid
1.	The first letter should be A, B, F, or M
2.	The second letter should be the same as the first letter of the prescriber's last name
3.	Add the first, third, and fifth numbers
4.	Add the second, fourth, and sixth numbers
5.	Multiply the answer from step 4 by 2
6.	Add the amount from step 5 to the amount from step 3
7.	The last number in this answer should be the same as the last digit of the DEA number

Example:
  Dr. James Hensley
  DEA number: AH2496570
  Is the DEA number valid?
Step 1: Is the first letter A, B, F, or M? YES
Step 2: Is the second letter the same as the prescriber's last name? YES
Step 3: 2 + 9 + 5 = 16
Step 4: 4 + 6 + 7 = 17
Step 5: 17 × 2 = 34
Step 6: 34 + 16 = 50
Step 7: Is the last number the same as the last digit in the DEA number? YES—the number is VALID.

SCHEDULE I NARCOTICS

. . . .

SCHEDULE II NARCOTICS

. . . .

SCHEDULE III NARCOTICS

Controlled Level	Schedule I (C-I)
Abuse potential	Has no accepted medical use in the United States (for research purposes only)
Examples	• crack cocaine • ecstasy • heroin • LSD • marijuana

Controlled Level	Schedule II (C-II)
Abuse potential	Has high potential for abuse
Examples	• Adderall® (amphetamine with dextroamphetamine salts) • Demerol® (meperidine) • Dilaudid® (hydromorphone) • Oxycontin® (oxycodone) • Percocet® (oxycodone with acetaminophen) • Ritalin® (methylphenidate)
Restrictions	No refills Cannot be phoned in except for emergencies

Controlled Level	Schedule III (C-III)
Abuse potential	Less potential for abuse then C-II
Examples	• Tylenol 3 (acetaminophen with codeine phosphate) • anabolic steroids
Restrictions	Can only be refilled a maximum of 5 times within 6 months

PHARMACY TECHNICIAN FLASH REVIEW

SCHEDULE IV NARCOTICS

. . . .

SCHEDULE V NARCOTICS

. . . .

DEA FORM 222

PHARMACY TECHNICIAN FLASH REVIEW

Controlled Level	Schedule IV (C-IV)
Abuse potential	Less abuse potential than C-II and C-III
Examples	• benzodiazepines (Xanax®, Valium®, Ativan®) • Ambien® (zolpidem) • Lunesta® (eszopiclone) • Soma® (carisoprodol)
Restrictions	Refill restrictions same as C-III (can only be refilled a maximum of 5 times within 6 months)

Controlled Level	Schedule V (C-V)
Abuse potential	Lowest possible abuse potential
Examples	• Lomotil® (diphenoxylate with atropine) • Lyrica (pregabalin) • Cough syrups with codeine
Restrictions	Some states allow dispensing without a prescription (must be 18 and sign a log)

DEA form used for ordering C-II medications—must be completed by a pharmacist only.

DEA FORM 224

. . . .

DEA FORM 106

. . . .

DEA FORM 41

Pharmacies must submit this form to register with the DEA prior to dispensing controlled substances.

· ·

Form completed by a pharmacy in the event of a theft of a controlled substance. The pharmacy must notify the nearest DEA office and complete the form.

· ·

Form must be submitted for destruction of controlled substances in the event of damaged or outdated medications.

DEA FORM REVIEW TABLE

. . . .

CONTROLLED SUBSTANCES INVENTORY

. . . .

DRUG ENFORCEMENT ADMINISTRATION (DEA)

DEA Form	Purpose
222	Ordering and returning C-IIs
224	Registering with the DEA
106	Theft of controlled substance
41	Destruction of outdated or damaged controlled substances

. . . .

Inventory must be taken every two years (exact count on C-IIs and estimated on C-III–V), and records kept for minimum of 2 years.

. . . .

Agency created under the CSA to enforce all controlled substance laws of the United States.

DRUG LISTING ACT OF 1972

. . . .

NATIONAL DRUG CODE (NDC)

. . . .

ORPHAN DRUG ACT OF 1983

Drug Listing Act of 1972	
Purpose	• FDA assigned each drug a specific number to identify it: the National Drug Code (NDC) number

Number assigned to each drug by the FDA:

• first five numbers = drug manufacturer

• second four numbers = drug product

• third set of two numbers = package size

Orphan Drug Act of 1983	
Purpose	• Provide tax incentives and expedited review and approval to manufacturers producing drugs for serious or life-threatening diseases affecting less than 200,000 patients (**orphan drugs**)

ORPHAN DRUG

. . . .

DRUG PRICE COMPETITION AND PATENT TERM RESTORATION ACT OF 1984

. . . .

BRAND NAME

A drug that is used to treat a disease that affects less than 200,000 patients.

. . . .

Drug Price Competition and Patent Term Restoration Act of 1984	
Purpose	• To encourage creation of generic drugs by streamlining the approval process for generic drugs
	• To encourage creation of new brand name drugs by extending patent licenses

. . . .

Proprietary name given by a drug manufacturer and protected by a patent.

ABBREVIATED NEW DRUG APPLICATION (ANDA)

· ·

GENERIC DRUG

· ·

CHEMICAL NAME

Documentation required by the FDA for generic drug makers; requires generic drugs to demonstrate bioequivalence to the brand name product, but does not require the same testing and clinical trials.

. . . .

Comparable to the brand name product in strength, dosage form, and route of administration; must also demonstrate similar effectiveness and efficacy, but is not protected by a patent.

. . . .

A scientific name based on the structure of the chemical compound.

PRESCRIPTION DRUG MARKETING ACT OF 1987

. . . .

ANABOLIC STEROID CONTROL ACT OF 1990

. . . .

ANABOLIC STEROID

PHARMACY TECHNICIAN FLASH REVIEW

Prescription Drug Marketing Act of 1987	
Purpose	• Prohibits the reimportation of a drug into the United States by means other than by the manufacturer
	• Prohibits the sale of drug samples and the distribution of samples to anyone other than those who are licensed to prescribe them

. . . .

Anabolic Steroid Control Act of 1990	
Purpose	• Designated anabolic steroids as a C-III substance due to misuse by athletes

. . . .

Synthetic testosterone abused by athletes and regulated under the Anabolic Steroid Control Act; classified as a schedule III narcotic.

OMNIBUS BUDGET RECONCILIATION ACT OF 1990 (OBRA-90)

. . . .

COUNSELING

. . . .

DIETARY SUPPLEMENT HEALTH AND EDUCATION ACT OF 1994 (DSHEA)

Omnibus Budget Reconciliation Act of 1990 (OBRA-90)	
Purpose	• Any participant in a Medicaid reimbursement program must undergo drug utilization review (DUR) by the pharmacist. • Every patient must receive an offer to be counseled by the pharmacist. • Failure to do so can result in loss of Medicaid reimbursement.

Done by the pharmacist to communicate with a patient any questions regarding medication or warnings and precautions that should be addressed.

• **A technician must never counsel patients, but can ask whether a patient has any questions for the pharmacist.**

Dietary Supplement Health and Education Act of 1994 (DSHEA)	
Purpose	• Manufacturers of supplements are permitted to make claims not approved by the FDA, but they must still comply with purity and safety standards to protect patients and prevent adulteration.

HEALTH INSURANCE PORTABILITY AND ACCOUNTABILITY ACT OF 1996 (HIPAA)

. . . .

MEDICARE PRESCRIPTION DRUG, IMPROVEMENT, MODERNIZATION ACT OF 2003 (MMA)

. . . .

FDA MODERNIZATION ACT OF 2004

Health Insurance Portability and Accountability Act of 1996 (HIPAA)	
Purpose	• Protect patient confidentiality of medical records, including prescription history

Medicare Prescription Drug, Improvement, Modernization Act of 2003 (MMA)	
Purpose	• Also known as Medicare Part D, provides prescription drug coverage to patients eligible for Medicare

FDA Modernization Act of 2004	
Purpose	• Change label on prescription drugs from "Caution: Federal Law Prohibits Dispensing Without a Prescription" to "Rx Only"

COMBAT METHAMPHETAMINE EPIDEMIC ACT OF 2005

. . . .

AFFORDABLE CARE ACT OF 2010 (ACA)

. . . .

FOOD AND DRUG ADMINISTRATION (FDA)

PHARMACY TECHNICIAN FLASH REVIEW

Combat Methamphetamine Epidemic Act of 2005	
Purpose	• Monitor usage of products that can be used to produce methamphetamine: • pseudoephedrine, ephedrine, and phenylpropanolamine • 3.6 g per day product limit, and patients must show valid ID to obtain • Medications stored behind the counter

Affordable Care Act of 2010 (ACA)	
Purpose	• To increase access to healthcare for uninsured Americans • Universal healthcare coverage to be in effect by 2014 for all citizens of the United States

Under the U.S. Department of Health and Human Services; responsible for:

- new drug review and approval

- generic drug approval

- issuing drug recalls if needed

- OTC drug reviews

NATIONAL ASSOCIATION OF BOARDS OF PHARMACY (NABP)

. . . .

CENTERS FOR MEDICARE AND MEDICAID SERVICES (CMS)

. . . .

STATE BOARDS OF PHARMACY (BOP)

Represents all 50 state boards of pharmacy; has no regulatory authority.

. . . .

Oversees all Medicare and Medicaid services; establishes conditions for a facility to be reimbursed for any services provided.

. . . .

Oversees the practice of pharmacy in each state; defines all roles and duties of pharmacists and pharmacy technicians; can discipline when necessary.

LICENSURE

. . . .

REGISTRATION

. . . .

CERTIFICATION

Permission by the state board for an individual to practice in a given occupation; individual must demonstrate a minimum competency in order to practice.

· ·

Enrolling on a list created by the state board of pharmacy.

· ·

A voluntary process in which an organization recognizes that an individual has met specific standards required for certification. **The Pharmacy Technician Certification Board (PTCB) certifies technicians, and this is required for practice in some states.**

UNITED STATES PHARMACOPEIA (USP)

. . . .

USP CHAPTER <797>

. . . .

USP CHAPTER <795>

PHARMACY TECHNICIAN FLASH REVIEW

Sets official standards for all prescription and OTC drugs manufactured and sold in the United States; sets standards based on quality, purity, strength, and consistency of product.

. . . .

Chapter of USP dedicated to sterile compounding and requirements to help eliminate contamination of compounded sterile products (CSPs).

. . . .

Chapter of USP dedicated to nonsterile compounding.

DRUG RECALL

. . . .

CLASS I RECALL

. . . .

CLASS II RECALL

May be issued by the FDA to withdraw a drug from the market or issued voluntarily by the manufacturer in the case of contamination or other liability concerns.

. . . .

Probability exists that use of the product or drug will lead to serious adverse health events or death.

- Example: label mix-up of a lifesaving drug

. . . .

Probability exists that use of this product or drug may cause adverse health events that will be reversible or temporary.

- Example: a drug labeled with an understrength that is not a lifesaving drug

CLASS III RECALL

. . . .

LOT NUMBER

. . . .

THE JOINT COMMISSION (TJC)

Probability exists that the use of this product will most likely NOT cause an adverse health event

- Example: container defect, off taste or smell

. . . .

Number assigned by a manufacturer based on the batch when it was produced; allows tracking of a product so that it can be located in the event of a recall

. . . .

Formerly known as the Joint Commission on Accreditation of Healthcare Organizations (JCAHO); accredits hospitals and evaluates facilities based on patient care standards and patient safety

MEDWATCH

. . . .

POLICIES AND PROCEDURES MANUAL

. . . .

GLOVE FINGERTIP SAMPLING

PHARMACY TECHNICIAN FLASH REVIEW

Voluntary program run by the FDA that allows any healthcare professional or patient to report a serious adverse event associated with the use of a specific drug.

· ·

A manual with written instructions for the pharmacy staff (both technicians and pharmacists) on all operations within the pharmacy.

• must be updated regularly

• must be written in accordance with hospital, state, and federal policies

• Any revisions and/or changes to policies must be approved by the appropriate committee (usually P and T committee).

· ·

Used as a quality assurance tool for sterile compounding procedures.

• detects the presence of microorganisms on the fingertips of gloves if a sterile compounding technician is using poor aseptic technique practices

• An agar plate is used to detect the pathogens.

• should be completed on personnel prior to compounding CSPs and annually thereafter as a part of competency training

NONSTERILE COMPOUNDING

. . . .

STERILE COMPOUNDING

. . . .

COMPOUNDED STERILE PREPARATION (CSP)

Compounding includes altering a drug to a form that is not commercially available based on instructions from a licensed prescriber. It can include: changing the dosage form or delivery system (e.g., crushing tablets and mixing to form a liquid), altering the strength of a drug (e.g., if a pediatric formulation is not available), combining two or more active ingredients, or preparing a drug from bulk products.

Compounding nonsterile products does not have to be done under sterile conditions, and the compound will be administered in a method that is not parenteral. The most commonly produced nonsterile compounds are suspensions, solutions, ointments and creams, suppositories, and tablets or capsules.

. . . .

Sterile compounding requires sterile conditions, meaning freedom from any bacteria or microorganisms. This process is reserved for parenteral products, or those injected, but can also be used for compounding medications being instilled into the eye and inhaled into the lungs.

. . . .

Also known as compounded sterile product, any drug that is compounded under sterile conditions.

ASEPTIC TECHNIQUE

....

GARBING PROCESS

....

PERSONAL PROTECTIVE EQUIPMENT (PPE)

The process used to prepare CSPs; this technique is vital to avoid microbial contamination of the medication being compounded.

· ·

Process must be followed strictly to prevent contamination; when finished, remove items in reverse order.

Garbing order (assume scrubs are already worn):

1. shoe covers

2. hair cover

3. face mask (beard cover if necessary)

4. wash hands aseptically

5. disposable gown

6. eye shield (if necessary)

7. sterile gloves

· ·

Essential for infection control and to protect the technician from blood-borne pathogens as well as exposure to hazardous chemicals.

Includes:

- gloves to protect the hands

- masks and a respirator to protect the respiratory tract as well as the nose and mouth

- goggles to protect the eyes in the event of any splashing

- face shields

ISOPROPYL ALCOHOL 70% (IPA)

. . . .

BEYOND USE DATING

. . . .

pH

Used for disinfecting and cleaning several areas:

- work surfaces of compounding area

- tops of vials prior to needle puncture

- gloved hands when necessary

. . . .

The date after which a product must not be dispensed or used (expiration date); this is determined by the pharmacist based on when the product is prepared and its storage conditions.

. . . .

A measure of how acidic or basic a solution is; closer to 1 is more acidic, and closer to 14 is more basic. **Blood pH is 7.4, so IV solutions should try to stay close to that value or at least neutral (pH = 7).**

TONICITY

. . . .

HYPERTONIC SOLUTION

. . . .

HYPOTONIC SOLUTION

PHARMACY TECHNICIAN FLASH REVIEW

How the cells in our body respond to surrounding fluid; three classifications—hypertonic, hypotonic, and isotonic.

. . . .

A solution that has **more** particles than the surrounding cells, which causes water to be drawn out of cells, and the cells to shrivel.

. . . .

A solution that has **fewer** particles than the surrounding cells, which causes water to be drawn into the cells, and the cells to swell and sometimes burst.

ISOTONIC

. . . .

COMPATIBILITY

. . . .

PHYSICAL INCOMPATIBILITIES

A solution that has **the same amount** of particles as the surrounding cells, so no water will move in or out, and the cell will stay the same size.

· ·

The ability to combine two or more products without creating a change in the physical, chemical, or therapeutic effectiveness of the drug.

· ·

When two or more drugs that are not compatible are combined, a physical change occurs that can be detected, including cloudiness, temperature, or a color change.

CHEMICAL INCOMPATIBILITIES

· ·

THERAPEUTIC INCOMPATIBILITIES

· ·

RISK LEVELS

When two or more drugs are combined and are not compatible, a chemical change occurs that may alter the pH of a solution or cause the decomposition of a component.

. . . .

When two or more drugs are combined that are not compatible, it causes a change in the effectiveness of one or more of the drugs when administered.

. . . .

Four contamination risk levels defined by the USP Chapter <797> include:

- low-risk CSPs

- medium-risk CSPs

- high-risk CSPs

- immediate-use CSPs

Assigned according to the probability of contaminating a CSP.

PHARMACY TECHNICIAN FLASH REVIEW

LOW-RISK CSPs

....

MEDIUM-RISK CSPs

....

HIGH-RISK CSPs

Involves the mixing of no more than three sterile products within an ISO class 5 workbench.

- Example: single transfer of a dosage from a vial into an IV bag

. . . .

Involves more complex sterile compounding procedures than low risk, such as mixing more than three sterile products or administering to multiple patients.

- Example: preparation of total parenteral nutrition (TPN)

. . . .

Involves mixing more than three products and/or one of the products is not sterile or is being compounded in an environment less than ISO class 5; these products must be sterilized before being injected into the patient.

- Example: using a nonsterile ingredient in preparing a medication for a patient

PHARMACY TECHNICIAN FLASH REVIEW

IMMEDIATE USE CSP

....

ANTEROOM

....

CLEAN ROOM

Intended to be used only for emergency situations or when a patient requires the immediate use of a CSP; must be administered within one hour of preparation.

Example: emergency medications for cardiopulmonary resuscitation

· ·

Area where pharmacy personnel prepare for sterile compounding, including:

- garbing

- hand washing

- gathering supplies

· ·

Place where hoods are housed to be used during sterile compounding; personnel should not enter unless properly garbed.

INTERNATIONAL ORGANIZATION FOR STANDARDIZATION (ISO)

. . . .

HIGH-EFFICIENCY PARTICULATE AIRFLOW FILTER (HEPA)

. . . .

HORIZONTAL LAMINAR AIRFLOW WORKBENCH (LAFW)

PHARMACY TECHNICIAN FLASH REVIEW

System for describing the maximum number of particles in the air allowed in a room where sterile products are compounded.

ISO Class	Maximum Particle Count (in particles of 0.5 microns and larger per m³ of air)
4	352
5	3,520 (minimum for compounding area of sterile products)
6	35,200
7	352,000 (minimum for clean rooms)
8	3,520,000 (minimum for anterooms)
9	35,200,000

Used to minimize airborne contamination by filtering 99.97% of particles sized 0.3 microns and greater.

A hood used to prepare CSPs that are not hazardous.

- Air is pulled into the hood through a prefilter and then filtered through the HEPA filter before blowing horizontally across the work surface toward the worker.

- Technicians must work 6 inches inside the hood to avoid mixing the unfiltered air of the clean room with the HEPA filtered air of the LAFW.

CLEANING THE HORIZONTAL LAWF

....

VERTICAL LAMINAR AIRFLOW WORKBENCH

....

SYRINGE

Must be cleaned at the beginning of each shift, before every batch compounding session, and if there are any major spills or cleanup of contaminated products.

Cleaning should be first done with sterile water to remove any residue, and then disinfected with 70% IPA.

- Start with the hood's hang bars and hooks.
- Next, clean the ceiling using overlapping motions starting from the back and moving toward the front.
- Next, clean the back of the hood starting from the top and moving back and forth to the bottom.
- Next, clean each side using down and up movements starting from the back of the hood to the exterior portion.
- Finally, clean the work surface starting from the back and using overlapping movements to clean until the front is reached.
- Be careful to not spray disinfectant on the surfaces, but rather on the cloth used to do the cleaning—this will protect the HEPA filter from absorption of chemicals.

· ·

A hood used to prepare CSPs that are hazardous (e.g., chemotherapy).

- Air flows down through the HEPA filter and is forced upward and vented outside.
- Technicians should wear eye protection and use double gloves for these preparations.

· ·

Used in the preparation of a CSP to withdraw or inject solutions.

Parts of a syringe:

- barrel—covered with calibration marks to measure fluid volume
- plunger—fits inside barrel; is moved in and out to adjust fluid volume
- tip—where the needle attaches; can be Luer-lock or slip-tip
  - Luer-lock: a secure connection with the needle and the syringe
  - slip-tip: the needle slides onto the syringe—not as secure
- Flat knob—end of the plunger, which is pulled to increase volume in the barrel

Special Precautions: The syringe can only be handled on the barrel or the flat knob; all other surfaces, if touched, can subject the medication to contamination.

NEEDLE

....

NEEDLE GAUGE

....

SHARPS CONTAINER

Used to puncture containers of medication and to withdraw or inject fluid. Parts of a needle:

- hub—end point that will attach to the syringe

- shaft—length of the needle

- bevel—slanted opening of the needle

- lumen—hollow portion of the needle where fluid moves

. . . .

The size of a needle is determined by its gauge.

- The higher the gauge, the smaller the opening or diameter (lumen) of the needle.

- The lower the gauge, the larger the opening or diameter of the needle.

- Ranges in size from 16-gauge to 25-gauge:
  - Example: A 16-gauge needle makes a larger hole than a 25-gauge needle.

. . . .

A red container used to safely dispose of all items considered dangerous and sharp, such as: needles, syringes, and broken glass.

VIAL

· ·

AMPULE

· ·

FILTER NEEDLE

A container that is sealed containing medication either in liquid or powder form.

- can be made from plastic or glass

- has a hard plastic cap that is removed by the technician prior to puncture

- can be either single-dose (preservative-free and can only be used one time) or multiple-dose (contains preservatives and is stable for up to 28 days from initial use)

· ·

A sealed container made from glass that has an elongated neck.

- must be broken prior to use

- Contains no preservatives—single use only

Opening an ampule:

- Make sure the medication is at the body (gently tap the head if necessary).

- Swab 70% IPA around the neck.

- Snap the neck away from you using gentle but firm pressure.

· ·

A needle used to withdraw fluid from an ampule; has a built-in filter to remove any glass particles that may have fallen into the medication.

LARGE VOLUME PARENTERAL

. . . .

SMALL VOLUME PARENTERAL

. . . .

IV SOLUTIONS

An IV infusion of greater than 250 mL (most commonly given as 500 mL or 1000 mL).

- used for electrolyte replacement and hydration
- given as a continuous infusion or IV drip

· ·

A CSP given usually as an IVPB over a short period of time.

- less than 250 mL (usually 150, 100, 50, or 25 mL)
- examples: antibiotics, antifungals, antiviral medications

· ·

Common IV Base Solutions	Also Known As
0.9% Sodium Chloride (NaCl)	Normal Saline (NS)
0.45% Sodium Chloride (NaCl)	0.45% Normal Saline (1/2 NS)
Lactated Ringer's	LR
Dextrose 5% in Water	D_5W
Dextrose 10% in Water	$D_{10}W$
Sterile Water for Injection	SWFI
5% Dextrose in 0.9% Sodium Chloride	D_5NS
5% Dextrose in 0.45% Sodium Chloride	$D_51/2NS$

DILUENT

. . . .

CORING

. . . .

TOTAL PARENTERAL NUTRITION (TPN)

A liquid used to reconstitute a powder medication before it is injected into a patient or another IV solution.

Common diluents:

- sterile water

- normal saline

· ·

The accidental introduction of small pieces of rubber from the top of a vial into the solution of medication; if this occurs, must discard vial.

· ·

An IV solution that provides nutrients for patients who are unable to eat or cannot get the nutrition they need through eating orally.

Composed of:

- sterile water (hydration)

- dextrose (sugar and carbs)

- amino acids (protein building blocks)

- lipids (fatty acids)

- electrolytes and other additives (vitamins and minerals)

- medications that a patient may need

COMPOUNDING LOG

. . . .

CLASS III PRESCRIPTION BALANCE

. . . .

PHARMACEUTICAL WEIGHTS

Used to record all entries of each compounded prescription so a reference can be available and easily accessible.

Lists the following information:

- date of compound
- Rx number
- names of specific ingredients used, along with:
  - expiration date
  - lot number
  - manufacturer
  - NDC number
- amount weighed or measured
- name of compound
- procedures detailing how compound was prepared
- name of preparer and pharmacist checking

. . . .

A two-pan balance that has a capacity of 15 to 120 grams.

- can be used to weigh small amounts in the range of +/– 5 mg
- used with pharmaceutical weights
- Weighing paper is placed on pans to prohibit contact of medication with the balance.
- Weighing boat can be used to weigh a larger quantity of a chemical.

. . . .

Weights used for calibration of class III prescription balance and for weighing ingredients.

- must be handled with forceps to avoid the transfer of any oils or dirt from the hands

DIGITAL BALANCE

· ·

GRADUATED CYLINDER

· ·

BEAKER

Uses one pan and a digital or analytical readout for weighing ingredients.

- easier to use than a class III balance and more accurate

. . . .

A glass or plastic tool used for measuring liquid volumes.

- range in size from 5 mL to more than 1,000 mL

- For highest degree of accuracy, always choose the smallest size that can measure the volume desired (e.g., choose a 100 mL cylinder to measure 95 mL—don't choose a 250 mL cylinder).

. . . .

Can also be used to measure larger volumes of liquid, but less accurate than a graduated cylinder.

MENISCUS

. . . .

MORTAR AND PESTLE

. . . .

OINTMENT SLAB

Curve at the upper surface of a liquid caused by surface tension.

- The liquid at the **bottom** of the meniscus should be measured at eye level.

· ·

Used in nonsterile compounding to grind substances.

Mortar—bowl-shaped item

Pestle—used for crushing or grinding substances

· ·

A flat surface used for mixing compounds such as creams, ointments, pastes, or gels.

- Usually made from ground glass, so it is nonabsorbent.

GEOMETRIC DILUTION

. . . .

TRITURATION

. . . .

LEVIGATION

A method that ensures equal distribution of ingredients:

- First, mix the ingredient in the smallest amount with an equal amount of the next ingredient in quantity.

- Mix these thoroughly, then add another amount equal to that which is now in the mortar and mix again.

- Continue this process, increasing in quantity until all ingredients are mixed evenly.

• •

Grinding tablets or other substances into a fine powder.

• •

A levigating agent is added to a triturated powder slowly to make a paste. Examples of levigating agents:

- mineral oil

- castor oil

- vegetable oil

- glycerin

SPATULATION

. . . .

PUNCH METHOD

. . . .

CAPSULE SIZES

PHARMACY TECHNICIAN FLASH REVIEW

Combining substances using a spatula.

· ·

A method for hand-filling capsules.

- The powder to be filled is placed on a surface, and the capsule is punched into the powder repeatedly until full.

· ·

Sizes range from 5 (smallest) to 000 (largest).

NOTES

NOTES

NOTES

NOTES